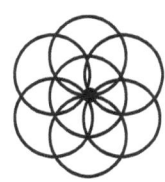

Sacred Steps

A Program for Soul Progression

based on

Ancient Yoga and A Course in Miracles

Bette Jean Cundiff

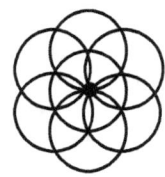

Miracle Experiences and You Publishing

You may contact the publisher and author at the following:

www.miracleexperiences.blogspot.com

bette@bettejeancundiff.com

ISBN-13: 978-1461178309

ISBN-10: 1461178304

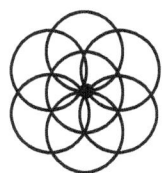

"There is a course for every teacher of God. The form of the course varies greatly. So do the particular teaching aids involved. But the content of the course never changes. Its central theme is always "God's Son is guiltless, and in his innocence is his salvation."

A Course in Miracles

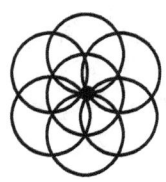

TABLE OF CONTENTS

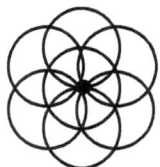

FORWARD

In *A Course in Miracles* our Elder Brother reminds us that there are no accidents.

*"There are **no accidents** in salvation.*
Those who are to meet will meet because together
they have the potential for a holy relationship.
They are ready for each other."

~*A Course in Miracles-original edition [ACIM-oe] Manual For Teachers #3 What are the Levels of Teaching?*

You have this book in your hands or you are reading it as an eBook and that is no accident. Every decision you have ever made throughout your entire life has brought you to this beautiful moment of NOW. And in this beautiful moment of NOW there is no past. The future is not yet. There is only this Holy Instant in which you are being called once again to LISTEN. LISTEN within for Guidance. LISTEN to your Soul and let it tell you the next right step on your journey without distance. That next right step may very well be these "***Sacred Steps***".

I first met Bette Jean Cundiff in New York City in the 1980's when I attended a workshop she was giving together with Paul Steinberg. Paul was the brother of Saul Steinberg who was the printer of the very first set of the hardback edition of *A Course in Miracles* through Coleman Graphics. The workshop was called, "Miracle Experiences: The Goals and Healing of Your Special Relationships in 'A Course in Miracles' " and was one of the first I had taken as I began my journey with *A Course in Miracles*.

Bette had also written "The Children's Material" which I used as a guide in bringing up my young son using the principles of *A Course in Miracles*. I owe Bette a debt of gratitude for this material and the benefit my son and I received. I recall my son would turn to me and in his little voice would childe me saying, "Mommy. Where is your happiness?"; Knowing I would remember that it is inside me, and would point to my own heart as we would both smile in remembrance and recognition. ♥

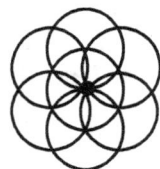

And now we come to "**Sacred Steps: A Program for Soul Progression**," Bette's most current book which appears to be a culmination of the past 30 years of studying, sharing, teaching and writing about what she has learned and what has been 'given' to her through inner Guidance.

As a student and teacher of Yoga, as well as a student of *A Course in Miracles*, I cherish the beautiful and artful integration of ancient yoga with A Course in Miracles that Bette presents here. The ideas are thought provoking and creative but more than that, they are presented in a way that brings a feeling of peace and unconditional love. I felt nurtured and safe and my heart opened to their Truth. The words were more like notes in a symphony and each word and even each letter seemed to be wrapped in LOVE; a LOVE which was almost palpable.

Describing each Chakra, Bette uses color, texture, and feeling to paint an in-depth picture offering a deep experience of their meaning. Then, in-between each description, additional information builds a foundation: Your Electromagnetic Field; The Power of the Universe as the Sacred Serpent; The Body's Windows [major organs and glands] ; The Earth's Windows [vortices]; The Celestial Radiance [personal aura]; The Rhythm of Color [Color as waves of energy]. I discovered that this foundation brought with it an appreciation for life.

"…And every time you walk into a room you change the whole electromagnetic energy field by your simple presence." P38

As well as a sense of renewed responsibility:

"*Your personal and radiant aura offers your message of peace and love to the world. It surrounds, you, caresses you and gently or powerfully touches the people in your life.*" P54

Bette beautifully presents the chakras as related to the levels of Soul evolution but then offers various modalities such as Sacred symbols [geometrics] as well as movement and affirmations to help with the integration. And finally there is practical application with a personal training program offered in the form of a Workbook.

My sense is that this book is a blessed gift offered to your Soul from another aspect of the Infinitude which is One with you. It's truly a gift of Love to Love. There is only this Holy Instant in which you are being called once again to LISTEN. LISTEN within for Guidance. LISTEN to your Soul and let it tell you the next right step on your journey without distance. That next right step may very well be these "*Sacred Steps*".

Reja Janaki Joy Green
Course in Miracles Society [CIMS]
Omaha, NE

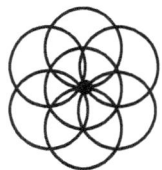

INTRODUCTION

"The Host of God has called to you, and you have heard."

A Course in Miracles

Your steps continue on the pathway Home. No one comes this far without an awareness of the journey he takes. The years roll by, lifetimes unfold, opportunities present themselves gain. Each instant becomes another glorious lesson filled with the learning of the ages, reflecting the wisdom of eternity.

You have begun to open your eyes to the wonder of your spiritual progress. No more are you blind to the deeper purpose of life in this world. But now a rich, 'new' meaning shapes every moment, every action, every encounter.

You have been called. . .and you have answered!

The following pages will cover lifetimes of study—study that has been accomplished through the journeys of many seekers over life after life, challenge after challenge, reward after reward. Thus, the Sacred Steps Study Program reflects the insights I have gained and the learning I have received from my travels into ancient yoga philosophies, comparative religions, co-dependency recovery -- And of course, from the more than thirty years of my studying and teaching the in depth spiritual psychology offered in the book entitled "A Course in Miracles."

In order for each of us to be a powerful light, a pocket of power in the dark and pain filled world, we must be able to clearly hear and then follow the Loving Direction that is within us. Within these pages you will find an overview of the journey we all must take to remembrance of our spiritual birthright, as well as easy step by step practices that will enhance your ability to follow any discipline and pathway on which you already walk.

Sacred Steps becomes, then, a power tool for opening, balancing and empowering

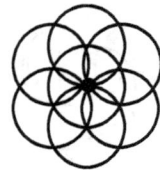

your energy centers and awakening the Holy Spirit, also called the kundilini that resides resting and waiting to flow powerfully through you. This is your program, designed over the millenniums, yet in the language of today. You and this program have evolved and met at just this perfect point in time and space.

May you follow these Sacred Steps to open you mind, fill it with light and speed your journey Home.

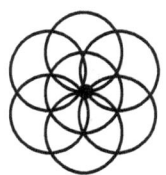

Alpha to Omega

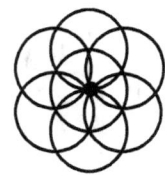

"The journey the Son of God has set himself is useless indeed,

but the journey on which his Father sets him is one of release and joy. . .

. . . when you reach its end it will roll up like a long carpet

spread along the past behind you, and will disappear. . ."

A Course in Miracles

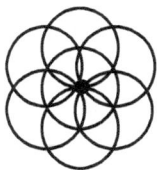

Time moves on and our lives are constantly changing. Nothing seems sure and firm. I take comfort watching the flow of the seasons, the cycles that nature gracefully follows - a dance of rising high in spring, twirling through summer, leaning and slowing in fall, and stretching out to rest in winter. And then the dance begins once more. My life from day to day and year to year from beginning to seeming end follows this dance as does yours. And so too, is seems, does the Universe. Here is a tale of this dance, if you wish, but one told by wise men throughout the ages that speaks of unimaginable lengths of time called Yugas.

From out of the vast stillness, the Essence of God, comes the outer expression of His creative Thought. There are as many different explanations of why and how this occurs as there are philosophies in the world to discuss this . . . and yet one theme weaves its way through them all. Beyond time and space, beyond the idea of form lies the realm containing the thought, the desire and the passion of Life. Here the journey begins and here it will ultimately end. In this realm of timeless being Life begins its journey to awareness. Here mind decides and develops, desires and designs. Here the beginning of expression will 'leave' the mind to wander in projected dreams through waves of black velvet moving across vast darkness. First, here is quiet, rest and waiting. Here in this place in mind all IS mind and thought is still.

Perhaps there is a stirring! A sudden pause in the stillness occurs. A small intense, almost painfully sharp insistence might begin to stab at the mind. A restlessness and a sense of need somehow is born. Though unknown before, an inner aching begins to grow nibbling from the center of mind 'outward'. The obsession grows and restlessness creates a yearning to find and bring to it that special something that can still its restlessness once more. Time is born--for now the time has come to begin the search for understanding and the remembrance of Home.

Thus, from the reality of formless Spirit comes a flow of experiences splintering and devolving into manifestation and then evolving once more to the remembrance of spiritual essence. A devolving and evolving from Alpha back to Omega, beginning to end.

In our next section we will explore a condensation of this devolving and evolving process using the symbol of a clock; and we will count off the cycle of Alpha to Omega in fifteen minute intervals. From the first thrust outward of consciousness to its reintegration and dissolution into the essence of God once more, we will travel around the Universe in 60 minutes.

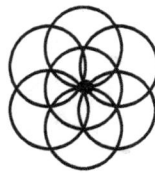

The Universe in 60 Minutes

"Can you imagine what it means to have no cares, no worries, no anxieties, but merely to be perfectly calm and quiet all the time? Yet that is what time is for; to learn just that and nothing more." A Course in Miracles

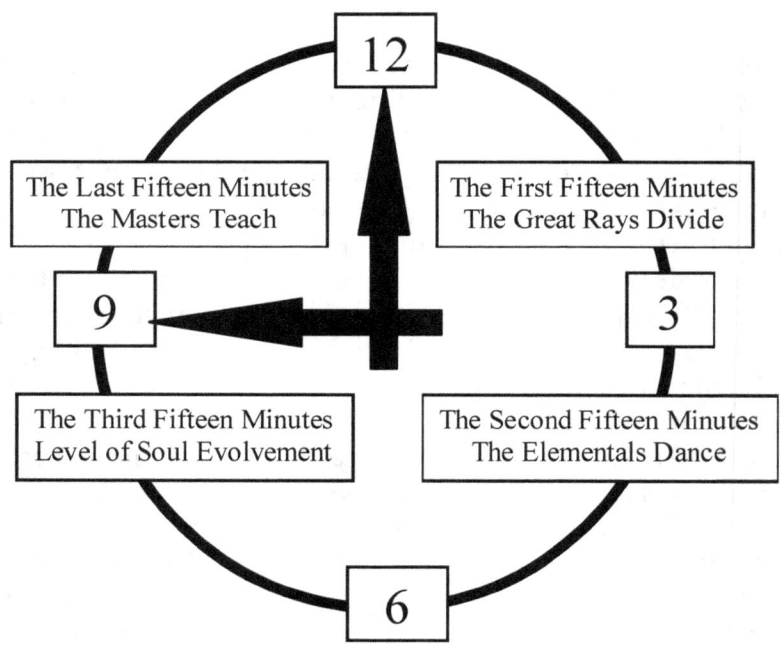

Tick, Tock, Tick, Tock….relentlessly this quiet sound continued as I rested this morning with my arms behind my head and my watch near my ear. Thoughts, feelings, memories marched by keeping time second by second to my ticking watch. And so, too, I contemplated, does all of life, only seasons are counted in months, human lifetime in years, -- but what of the whole Universe?

The most ancient of teachings, the Vedas, suggests Brahma breaths out and the universe forms, then breaths in and the universe disappears. And this continues eternally through Infinity. Let's take a take a look at one full breath, or Yuga, as if it were the sixty minutes that show on the face of my watch.

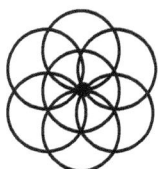

The First Fifteen Minutes

"In many only the spark remains, for the Great Rays are obscured. Yet God has kept the spark alive so that the Rays can never be completely forgotten. If you but see the little spark you will learn of the greater light, for the Rays are there unseen."
A Course in Miracles

The first division occurs with the outflowing of thought. The expression of God's mind seems to divide once, twice and so on until the first seven expressions are formed. This is the Light of God, focused through the prism of limitation creating the Seven Great Rays. Now each Ray will represent certain aspects of creation:

The first three Rays:
  1 - Will and Power - Life Force
  2 - Love and Wisdom - Compassion
  3 - Intelligence and Activity - Guidance
The last four Rays:
  4 - Harmony and Beauty - will devolve into Art
  5 - Concrete Knowledge - will devolve into the Sciences
  6 - Devotion and Prayer - will devolve into Religions
  7 - Ceremony and Ritual - will devolve into Politics/Economics

As these Rays shine down they begin to divide again and again creating a kaleidoscoping and spinning chaos of energies and potentials that will eventually evolve into manifestation in the world as we experience it. But for now the first fifteen minutes are complete.

The Second Fifteen Minutes

"The world of perception, on the other hand, is the world of time, of change, of beginnings and endings." A Course in Miracles

Energies swirl and dance like dervishes, dividing and gathering once more. Here the "elementals" play. Here rhythms of fragmented thoughts jumble together. They dance to a tune still discordant and not yet fully developed. These elemental energies will become the building blocks to matter, the matter that will form the universe we know. But for now they are only a misty shadow of what will be. Dark and ominous, as well as playful and frivolous these elementals are the underlying vibration of physical manifestation.

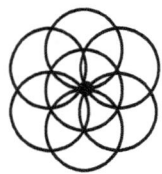

As we get closer to the ending of the first half hour these elemental energies seem more familiar. We can recognize them in our dreams as goblins and gremlins, fairies and nature spirits. These varied energies are the foundation from which our minds will eventually create the concrete physical world.

But now time continues onward and the rumblings of the dance become stronger, the movements of the elementals more frantic. An excitement builds to crescendo proportions. The dance comes to its climax - an explosion of light and sound and FORM appears! The "bang" of creation is heard for the first time and expansion forms a universe filled with gases and stars, planets and meteors. The half hour is complete and the stage is set for humanity to appear and life to evolve upward.

The Third Fifteen Minutes

". . .you have barely started to allow your first
uncertain steps to be directed up the ladder separation led you down."
A Course in Miracles

The universe has devolved to the farthest point away from the Pure Thought of God. Formless Spirit is forgotten in a seeming concrete dream. And now humanity begins its first tentative steps up the ladder of evolution. As this second half hour continues humanity begins the spiraling journey to remembrance. From these first efforts, barely removed from the elemental Dance, the myths and legends of half beast half man, giants and lands of magic and fantasy unfold. The planets are still forming also, and so the kingdoms of mineral, plant animal and man parallel each other on their journey upwards.

As time moves through these fifteen minutes humanity becomes more recognizable and incarnational cycles begin. Each lifetime now gives opportunities for lessons on life and love. Seven distinct vibrational classrooms of learning, must be traversed. We may call them the Levels of Soul Evolvement and will study them more closely and in greater depth in the following section. Each of these classrooms offers a field of growing power and responsibilities. Just like climbing a mountain, each step up the incarnational spiral is demanding, perhaps exhausting and yet each step brings a view of life that is clearer and more panoramic the higher you proceed.

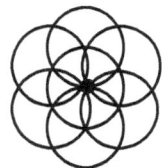

As humanity climbs this mountain each person's accomplishments become a safety harness protecting those who follow. The lessons, clothed in varied experiences are one - to love all and share an understanding of this oneness. As humanity, one by one, completes this lesson, each becomes a transcended Master and enters the next fifteen minutes.

The Last Fifteen Minutes

". . .in time it can be said that the advanced teachers of God
have the following characteristics. . ."
A Course in Miracles

Love lights this realm. Here the Masters teach. Here they have recognized their oneness and become the shared identity of the metaphysical Christ. They also recognize that there are so many other Souls yet to learn this blessed lesson.

Within these last fifteen minutes the transcended Masters, who have evolved through the spiraling incarnations of the third fifteen minutes, continue to be of service. Time is running out and every Soul must be helped up the mountain and around the final half hour to Omega. These Masters send their understanding down into the minds of the evolving Souls below. They offer the awareness of oneness, as well as the practical advice necessary to attain this awareness.

Occasionally a Master will visit the final stage of the previous fifteen minutes. Though he no longer need journey there he can choose to stay for a short while should the vision of his presence be of help. He becomes one of history's avatars.

These final fifteen minutes collapse very quickly. As more and more Souls enter this final time period of awareness and service the evolving souls below are drawn up more quickly literally sucked by the growing power. As the light of each soul gathers together with others into the seven major colors of the Great Rays, these Rays then condense once more into the brilliance of God's Radiance and Alpha becomes Omega. Time ends and only God remains.

In the next section, let's focus closely on just the third fifteen minutes, which I have labeled the Levels of Soul Evolovement, and follow the step by step evolving Soul through its many lifetimes.

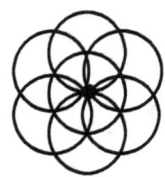

The Scale
of
Soul Evolvement and Actualization

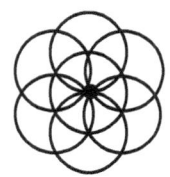

Scale of Soul Evolvement

How far you have evolved and in which level you are functioning.

Scale of Actualization

How much learning you are using.

Transcendence to Hierarchy and MASTER LEVEL   *Pure Thought Energy*

...... 80.0

700 ALPHA to OMEGA Divine Principle Incarnate

Energy Flows through the Crown Portal
Body Used at will
Mind ⟩ *Seen as one*
Spirit

| 799 |
| 701 |

Your learning ends here though you may return to be a Master teacher

Mastery

...... 70.0

600 THE KNOWER Illuminated

Energy Flows through the Forehead Portal   **FOCUS** Cosmic Will
Body Gaining detachment   **IDEAL** Universal Connectedness
Mind Gaining Cosmic Consciousness   **EXPLORATION** Inner Universes
Spirit Opening to Nirvana

| 699 |
| 665 |
| 635 |
| 601 |

Inner worlds become more important than outer

...... 60.0

Transition (590-610) Relinquishing old, transiting to new -Emotional and disorienting

500 ACCEPTED DISCIPLE Achievement in Service

Energy Flows through the Throat Portal   **FOCUS** Teaching Cosmic Principles
Body Recognition of illusion   **IDEAL** World Teacher
Mind Learning Cosmic Identification   **EXPLORATION** Innovative Service
Spirit Full Trust of Spiritual Guidance

| 599 |
| 565 |
| 535 |
| 501 |

Utilizing greater power in the public arena

........50.0

Transition (490-510) Relinquishing old, transiting to new -Emotional and disorienting

400 PROBATIONARY DISCIPLE Introduction to Spiritual Commitment

Energy Flows through the Heart Portal   **FOCUS** Teacher of spirituality
Body Tool for service   **IDEAL** Service through ministry
Mind Learning mental control   **EXPLORATION** Spiritual Pathways
Spirit Learning to work with the Hierarchy

| 499 |
| 465 |
| 435 |
| 401 |

Beginning to express personal charisma

...... 40.0

Transition (390-410) Relinquishing old, transiting to new - emotional and disorienting

300 ASPIRANT Developing Mind

Energy Flow through the Solar Plexus Portal   **FOCUS** Intellect
Body Secondary to the mind   **IDEAL** Mind power
Mind Scholarly pursuit   **EXPLORATION** Data/information
Spirit Touched by the Hierarchy

| 399 |
| 365 |
| 335 |
| 301 |

Accepting greater responsibility
More stable emotionally

• 30.0

Transition (290-310) Relinquishing old, transiting to new - emotional and disorienting

200 PILGRIM Exploring the Physical World's Energy

Energy Flows through the Navel Portal   **FOCUS** Material Values
Body Learning dexterity   **IDEAL** Physical Perfection
Mind Task oriented/basic imagination   **EXPLORATION** Physical Universe
Spirit Superstition/God as Authority figure

| 299 |
| 265 |
| 235 |
| 201 |

Learning Spiritual Competency

...... 20.0

100 ENTITY Learning Existence

Energy Flows through the Root Portal of Power
Body Learning Survival Skills
Mind Undeveloped Reason
Spirit Feels a glimmer

| 199 |
| 165 |
| 135 |
| 101 |

You start here with your first lifetimes in a body

Denial of Addiction, Co-dependency
Little energy

.... 10.0

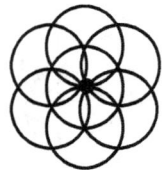

"Forget not once this journey is begun the end is certain."

A Course in Miracles

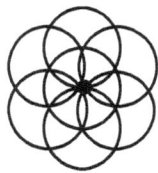

A discussion of the Levels of Soul Evolvement

We come, we go. We stretch, we grow. And so our Souls begin, continue and eventually end the cycles of reincarnation undoing past karma. This concept of repeated lives comes to us through the mists of time and is not unique nor attached to any one religion or philosophical system of study. From ancient times to the present humanity has demonstrated a collective sense of a continuum of experiences that seem to spiral to greater and greater levels of understanding. These levels can in fact be charted and measured by one attuned to the electromagnetic field of energy that streams forth from an individual's aura.

Take a look once more at the chart entitled "Scale of Soul Evolvement and Actualization". Reading from the bottom up you will notice seven distinct stages on the left side, The Levels of Soul Evolvement, representing the measurable levels of energy patterns of spiraling learning that all Souls progress through to final transcendence as a Master Teacher of the Spiritual Hierarchy. These seven levels have been consistently referred to in many of the books that discuss spiritual growth. I was introduced to a chart simpler than this in the late 1970's. Guidance directed me to add much more from Yoga Philosophy and so here I offer my unique system. I have labeled the levels according to my own research as well as from the voluminous experiences I gained while measuring the energy fields of thousands of people and then measuring the changes after working with the Sacred Symbols. (You will read about this amazing tool in the following chapters.) One of my dear friends, who I introduced to this work about that time, is Dr. David Hawkins who has 'run' with this concept in an exciting and stupendous way adding his own extensive pscyhiatric experiences to his work. *(He also graciously wrote the forward to my book, "Side by Side – the Twelve Steps and A Course in Miracles)*

In the previous pages we disucssed "The Universe in 60 Minutes". This section discussed "The **Third** Fifteen Minutes" offering a preliminary insight into The Levels of Soul Evolvement. These seven levels can be compared with different classrooms each offering a specific area for growth and learning. As you grow and advance you can only progress upwards, never backwards down the chart!

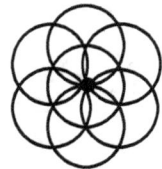

What you have learned you can never lose, but you can choose to decide not to use it! The Actualization Level seen on the right side of the chart, reflects the extent to which you are willing to apply all the knowledge you have gained so far. If you are using all the understanding available to you from all your karmic lessons gleaned over innumerable lifetimes your Soul number and your Actualization number will be in perfect balance, and will be directly across from each other on the chart.

I am often asked, "How many lifetimes does it take to complete a full level on the Scale for Soul Evolvement?" My answer is this: You will live as many lifetimes as is necessary to learn how to utilize that power field effectively and responsibly. Progress up the Scale proceeds slowly in the lower levels and speeds up through the higher levels. And so it may take anywhere from two to twenty lifetimes to complete a spiral through just one of the seven levels. Perhaps fifteen to twenty on the lowest, three to ten on the middle levels, and the last two may need only one major *push* each.

How many lifetimes does it take to learn to change a light bulb? I guess you have to learn how to create a light bulb first. This really, really small joke is a reminder that our evolving souls sure have to go through a lot to finally get to be at the Mastership level. Keep in mind: How open you are to spiritual guidance will determine how quickly and successfully you spiral upwards through the levels of Soul Evolvement, healing issues involving health, wealth and relationships. No one can go backward! All life experiences will stretch you. You will learn from them. How much you are willing to learn compassion, forgiveness and true spiritual detachment will determine the speed of your journey. But no one can stop completely or reverse the learning process; and each level on the scale is a vital, fulfilling and necessary classroom where you become both student and teacher!

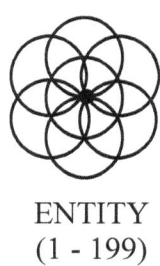

ENTITY
(1 - 199)

"Each time you practice, awareness is brought a little nearer at least; sometimes a thousand years or more are saved." A Course in Miracles

Classroom: Existence
Curriculum: Learning basic survival skills
Perspective: Childlike
Success: Survival
% of Population - .0005%

From 1 - 199 on the Scale of Soul Evolvement the beginning of a series of seeming unending lives unfold. Here breakthrough from the elemental energy to the physical plane of existence occurs. These births into the physical world are filled with shock, excitement and addictive pleasure. The Soul is sensing life in a totally new and exhilarating way. These first lifetimes are filled with great emotional confusion for they represent the first primitive use of the concrete world of form. Those Entities struggling through this energy field rely almost entirely on instinct and can succeed only through constant repetition of actions. They are driven by their emotions with almost no understanding of the underlying reasons for their lives and activities. Only a small percentage of people on the planet fall into this level. The majority of Souls are found stretching through the next range.

PILGRIM
(200 - 299)

"...(here) the toys and trinkets of the world are sought..."
A Course in Miracles

Classroom: Physical work, physical body, physical universe
Curriculum: Exploring sensuality, sexuality, power, money, physical prowess
Perspective: Spirituality expressed in dogmatism, religious symbols concrete (i.e. God is old man with beard), tends toward superstition
Success: Perfect body, material abundance, physical power
% of Population - 50%

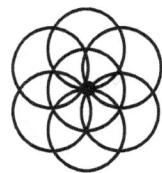

From 200 - 299 the Soul begins the adventure of learning to be an active participant in the physical world. Here is learned the rudimentary process of creating civilizations, the power of money, the varied possible uses and parameters of the physical body and the first glimpse of a Higher Power through superstition and the practice of ritual.

For those growing through the experiences of the Pilgrim the responsibility of handling money, treating relationships ethically, learning about basic health issues and reaching toward God through ritual and rigid dogma becomes a necessary series of challenges. Unlike education in our present society, no one can slip through the system and graduate without learning the lessons. But once learned, they cannot be forgotten. You can refuse to utilize them, but you can never be without them.

Felt the nudge of a Transcended Master lately? Well, that's what happens when you reach this next level of the Scale of Soul Evolvement. Let's take a look at this next level – Aspirant. You just may see yourself or those you know reflected in this description.

ASPIRANT
(300 - 399)

*"Helpers are given you in many forms. . .
for Christ takes many forms with different names
until their oneness is recognized."*
A Course in Miracles

Classroom: Mind
Curriculum: Philosophical, psychological and parapsychological development and exploration.   Accumulation, categorization and dissemination of information.
Perspective: Natural student and teacher acquiring and sharing information
Success: Being recognized as one of the most knowledgeable in one or more fields
% of Population - 20%

Our journey continues. During the previous two levels existence and survival were learned and then insight and strength in dealing with the basics of the physical world were added. Now begins the trek upward through the exploration of the mind!

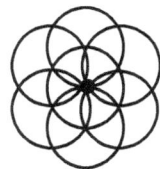

Before we continue, refer to the Scale of Soul Evolvement making note that all seven levels could be divided into three areas of growth. The lowest third of each level brings with it a great sense of excitement about the new adventures to unfold. This is the point of unknown territory never experienced before. The energies channeling through the first third of this classroom are strange and untested. You have not been here before. The world and what it offers, however, draws you onward as this plays on your unquenchable curiosity. On this level of Aspirant, during the first third of the level you begin to use your mind through a great ability to memorize details.

As you increase in power and energy you move upward into the next third of this level. The second third always offers the expanding Soul an opportunity to express fully the lessons taught in a particular classroom. As an Aspirant, at this point of growth, you explore mind and realize the great potential within it, and begin to push this to its limit. The natural psychic is born. This talent may not always be labeled, but is always felt as a deep intuition and sensitivity to the environment.. You begin to sense a greater meaning to life. You begin to see the woven tapestry of the Universe and the integrity of it all. You cannot but ask, "What is my part in all of this?"

This simple but profound question is asked again and again from now on. And it is not ignored! One Who can guide you to your fullest expression hears your call and begins to guide your mind. A transcended Master from the Spiritual Hierarchy, who has completed his own journey along the Scale of Soul Evolvement, feels your desire and will now be there to guide your footsteps. You may not understand this consciously but will always feel this. You have been recruited by the Hierarchy to work with them and you have the choice to accept. When you do accept, you cross the Scale at 375, a point of "no return".

As you enter upward into the final third of the level of Aspirant you become a natural teacher. All of the lessons you have accomplished over many lifetimes in just this level alone demand organization and dissemination. At this point you are ready to synthesize what you have learned and share this with others. This is a time of re-evaluating your mind and how it functions! You are being asked to throw away what has never really worked, as well as what has served you so far but needs updating. Before this you had a sense of success and competency, but in this final third of this level you begin to exhibit growing restlessness. You become bored with your job and career. You question how you are handling your relationships and begin to question deeply your purpose in life. You want to understand the why and how of all things. And in order to truly gain this wisdom you must give up most, if not all of what you have already learned!

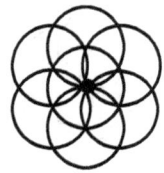

Special Numbers to keep in mind:

350   The desire to grow and learn increases. Opening to psychic experiences with an emphasis on the excitement and glamour.

365   Through hard work and diligence one becomes bright enough to be seen and approached by a transcended Master and recruited to be a disciple. The choice is offered to accept discipleship and acceleration into the 400's in this lifetime or to continue a slow evolution through the 300's for the rest of the lifetime.

375   Point of no return - a conscious agreement is made to work with the Hierarchy as a disciple and to accelerate through this level in this lifetime.

380's   Dress rehearsal for transition - a time of letting go marked be upheavals.

390's   Beginning of transition and a time of grief adjusting to all that must be lost in order to gain the rewards that are coming but not yet seen.

So your world feels like it's falling apart - and has been for quite a while? Things just keep being 'taken away', or so it seems. Has grief becomes a constant companion? Take heart, you asked for this. You made an inner commitment and transition from the present level to the next just 'ain't easy'!

Transitions Between Level

". . .a sense of actual disorienation may occur. But fear it not, for it means only that you have been willing to let go your hold on the distorted frame of reference that seeemed to hold your world together. . .The period of which precedes the actual transition, is far shorter than the time it took to fix your mind so firmly on illusions. . ."
A Course in Miracles

Thus begins the disorienting ending of this energy field. This time of transition from the 300's to the 400's begins at 390 and ends at 410 on the Scale of Soul Evolvement. From 390 to 400 you enter a dark tunnel. On a day to day basis you do not know where you are going, or even why! You find yourself losing things; perhaps your job, a relationship, or you must move from one city to another. It may even seem as if you are losing your mind!

This is a time for faith, for what you are really being asked to lose are your self-destructive habits and thinking processes. You are being asked to give up the old and

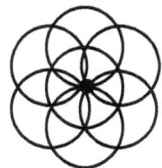

out grown and jump into the new. And your spiritual progress will be determined by your willingness to trust this process.

Remember, power is neutral. As you progress through transition into the next level greater and greater power will channel through you. Drag your bad habits along with you and they will gain greater power! Thus your responsibility toward yourself and others grows directly in proportion to the power you gain. Luckily, your understand is also growing proportionately!

PROBATIONARY DISCIPLE
(400 - 499)

"I am here only to be truly helpful,
I am here to represent Christ Who sent me. . ."
A Course in Miracles

Classroom: Spirituality
Curriculum: Exploring spiritual pathways and developing a personal ministry
Perspective: Growing personal charisma. Trusting inner guidance. Accepting a clear spiritual function and role
Success: Being a leader   % of Population - 15%

As you cross the 400 mark you enter the next level of learning on the Scale of Soul Evolvement. These first ten points, 400-410, will be the final part of transition. Then you will move into the excitement of new spiritual adventures. A sense of real purpose thrusts you into a greater and deeper exploration of spiritual studies. You have now become a Probationary Disciple of your transcended Master. And whether he is consciously known to you or not at this time he will be; and you will want to learn all you can about the pathway he directs you to, and which you will follow for the rest of your many, many lifetimes.

Your heart begins to open and you desire real forgiveness to enter your mind. How to accomplish all this is yet to be fully learned on this level and so you will find yourself drawn into relationships that can offer you the opportunity again and again to see this lesson at work in your life. During your sojourn on this level you may attempt to re-establish broken relationships disrupted by the preceding transition period. You may not have dropped all your old patterns, and so these affairs offer you the opportunity to once more give up out grown and now inappropriate behavior.

25

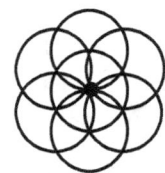

The desire to establish yourself with groups grows, for on the inner level you are feeling compelled to be of service to humanity and so will help form organizations toward this end. As you reach the middle of the level of Probationary Disciple your personal power and charisma will have increased impressively and you will be noticed by others. Your leadership unfolds naturally at this point and impacts powerfully on the group or organization you are with.

By the time you reach the final third of this level you will have made spiritual service a full time "job". Perhaps not as a job title in the marketplace, but certainly service to the world has become your full time focus.

Special numbers to keep in mind:

410 - 425	A time of new adventures, new relationships, new challenges
425 - 470	A natural establishment of leadership with clear focus and function
475	Point of no return - commitment to full time spiritual service

At this point you once more begin the disorienting transition of moving from 490 to 510. Now the choice is not whether you must give up behavior patterns disrupting your relationships, but to make a choice for the willingness to give up your value systems, across the board!

By now you probably have a general sense of where you have been and where may be on this chart. But are you ready to be truly masterful in this lifetime. Next we will look at what it takes to becoming masterful and the challenges specific to those levels. Remember, only a very few make this transition to the 500's . . . and beyond.

ACCEPTED DISCIPLE
(500 - 599)

"I am among the ministers of God."
A Course in Miracles

Classroom: Accepted Discipleship
Curriculum: Exploration of cosmic principles and recognition of illusion
Perspective: Work can become internationally known and become a legacy to humanity
Success: Spiritually innovative
% of Population - 10%

The Accepted Disciple is an innovator. From 500-599 on the Scale of Soul

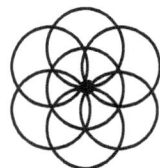

Evolvement you will have a burning desire to create anew! Up to now you have studied one or more established philosophies and been a teacher of these ideas. Perhaps you have even become a minister, or perhaps simply a leader for friends and co-workers. Now, however, your personal power has increased along with your integration of these studies. These talents create a formidable team and express powerfully through you into the world. You begin to work consciously with the Spiritual Hierarchy and your Master.

Your work through this level will be to give a new twist to old teachings. Your work can become internationally known. You may travel around the world giving your insights to thousands upon thousands yearning for understanding. Should your work be expressed in a more concrete way as books, music, works of art and scientific breakthroughs, it will last and be appreciated beyond your own lifetime and left as a legacy to humanity. Your power has now grown into worldly proportions.

Throughout this level you must still perfect the lessons of forgiveness in relationships. The constant challenge of doing your spiritual work within a work predominantly filled with Souls lower on the Scale and not yet ready to hear and accept what you have to offer may drain you. Only unbending faith in your Master and His guidance can support you through this level.

As you spiral to the end of this level of learning, you once more enter into transition. The choice is clear: Are you willing to give up all the privileges that come with being world renowned and become once more unknown? Should your answer be yes you move onto the next level.

Each transition period between levels is a form of "death". Many actually choose this time to give up their bodies between lifetimes. The reason is simple - in order to funnel the great amount of increasing energy and power through your body it must be up to the demand. Though the desire to continue your progress may be strong, you may have neglected the vehicle which you must use, your body. At each step up the spiraling ladder of spiritual progress you are given opportunities to improve your body as well as your mind. There are many pathways that offer specific methods for doing this and there is no one and only system. The one that will work for you and offer your body the greater actualization of its potential will be presented to you at the right time. It will be up to you to recognize it - and use it!

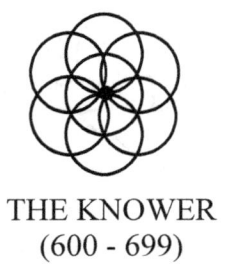

THE KNOWER
(600 - 699)

"And finally, there is a 'period of achievement.' It is here that learning is consolidated."
A Course in Miracles

Classroom: Knowing the Inner World
Curriculum: Exploration of inner world and universal connectedness through introspection
Perspective: Gaining detachment and cosmic unity
Success: Illumination
% of Population - 5%

What will be your purpose as a Knower? You must give up all labels placed on yourself and become naked before God. Your time must be spent predominantly in introspection. The "veils between dimensions" become extremely thin and you are able to consciously integrate the experience of being on several dimensions of existence at once. Now your work with the Hierarchy spans the physical dimension into the invisible.

Your outer work will still go on. Your family life continues normally as does your responsibility to them. This must never be ignored. Your lessons are still those of forgiveness. The major change has become your purpose. Listening to God in all ways and through all activities becomes your twenty-four hour a day activity. And so you progress from 600 to 699.

Wouldn't you love to think you are a walking Master, or can reach that level in this lifetime? Well, you have probably have had truly masterful moments, and that you can be proud of! But, that just isn't quite enough. Consistancy must be achieved, and that takes a really long, long time.

At this time in history, on the planet, few are at the point of completing the 600 level of the Knower, and only the rare individual will travel through the next transition into another incarnational cycle. Most will end their journey along the Scale of Soul Evolvment here, and will continue to learn, to grow and to be of help from other dimensions. From now on only a few volunteers will continue on up the Scale in physical form. They will become the avatars and messiahs and grace the world with their radiant presence.

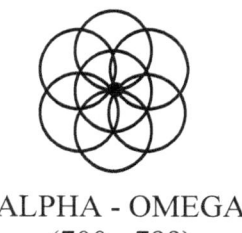

ALPHA - OMEGA
(700 - 799)

"These might be called the Teachers of teachers because
although they are no longer visible, their image can yet be called upon.
And they will appear when and where it is helpful for them to do so."
A Course in Miracles

Classroom: Divine Principle Incarnate
Curriculum: None - simply walking through the last of past karma
Perspective: Transcendent and complete union of all
Success: Simply Being
% of Population - Very few

Here walks the living Master. Though he too must continue to walk through his past karma in a seeming spiral of lessons on forgiveness, he does this with complete awareness and faith. Traveling up this final level will occur all in one lifetime. When one is born into this level the child bears within him the awareness of all his past lifetimes and the learning of trillions and trillions or more lessons. All is available to him consciously. He wields the greatest power and understands fully the responsibility that comes with its use.

These avatars and messiahs are only rarely recognized by others. The reason is obvious, for unless one is willing to open his heart and mind to the highest and most complete level of love offered by these masters, this vibrational energy will seem invisible. For most people, they simply will not see what they do not want to see or can believe.

There are also some transcended Masters who have completed the Scale of Soul Evolvement and who choose to appear for limited periods on the planet. They only visit for short times offering their image, thus giving added power and acceptability to their message and their guidance. They are not here for full lifetimes, but for just a quick 'guest' appearance.

And so here, at 799 the end of spiraling lessons occurs. Once this point is reached it is no longer necessary to return to physical form. Though some may choose to visit. Are there more lessons to learn beyond this last lifetime? Perhaps, but these lessons occur in a manner not to be understood by those of us who still must use time and form.

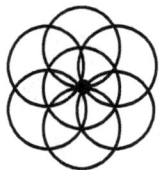

But for all, from the Entity just entering the spiral of reincarnational learning to the transcended Master continuing to bend down to the rest of humanity, the message and the lesson remain the same. . .

". . . take the time to love!"

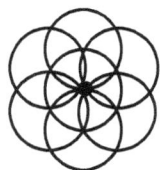

A Discussion of the
Levels of Actualization

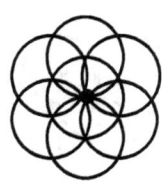

"The escape from darkness involves two stages.
First, the recognition that darkness cannot hide.
This step usually entails fear.
Second, the recognition that there is nothing you want to hide even if you could.
This step brings escape from fear."

A Course in Miracles

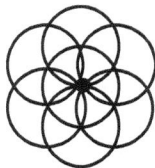

Are you feeling these symptoms?

"I know this, so why am I not doing it!"
"I have decisions to make, but I can't even discern the choices!"
"When I do make decision I have trouble following through."
"It seems life is mostly overwhelming and confusing"
"I seem to be facing life's challenges like a final exam. I have studied really hard, but have refused to eat or sleep before taking the test -- so I sabotage my efforts."

Sound familiar? Sure it does. That's because most of us may have traveled up the Scale of Soul Evolvement quite a ways, but we hang onto some unfortunate self-sabotaging habits. Let's take a further look at this phenomenon.

The Actualization Level reflects your growing spiritual maturity. It represents how much you are actually using of the accumulated learning that the Soul Level represents. Just because you know a whole lot about spirituality, does not necessarily mean you will utilize that information and understanding. Here is the difference between between 'talking the talk and walking the walk'. There are too many who fool themselves and as well as others into thinking they are much more accomplished than they are, simply because they sound so smart!

As you study the chart of Evolvement and Actualization, you can probably discover about how far you have evolved. Now, if you are fully using all your accumulated learning, you would then find your Level of Actualization directly across from your Level of Soul Evolvement. If your Soul number is measured at 350 and you are fully using all your past learning experiences, then your Actualization number would measure 35.0.

However, most individuals are usually out of balance with a much lower Actualization number than their Soul number, and this probably means you, also. Just take another look at the symptoms above and you will know this is true.

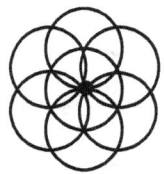

As you study the Actualization Levels on the previous chart of the Scales of Soul Evolvement and Actualization, here are some measurements to keep in mind:

under 18.0
Emotionally acting like an infant. Strong denial and refusing to deal with issues. Highly co-dependent and addictive.

19.0-20.0
Willingness for change grows and a desire to take responsibility and look within for correction.

20.0-30.0   **Learning steps to spiritual maturity:**

        Step 1 - Recognize breakdown areas in yourself immediately
        Step 2 - Label breakdown areas honestly and accurately
        Step 3 - Get ***appropriate*** help
        Step 4 - Follow through and learn to do things correctly. (This takes time!)

over   30.0
Getting closer to balancing both levels and is working with some spiritual or self-help program

over   35.0
Probably in balance or close to it (since so many of you reading this are proably in the high 300's or 400's.)

What about children?

Most children are born with a low Actualization measurement. Duh! Just observe any two year old, or for that matter any twelve year old. But take heart if you are a parent, as children physically mature they have the opportunity to also spiritually mature and bring their measurement up into balance. Here is where the parents can help out if they are evolving and balancing their own measurements.

Balance can be accomplished by the time a child reaches anywhere from sixteen to twenty-five years old. Sadly, however, they rarely do. In fact, most adults have fairly low Actualization measurements, way out of balance with their Soul measurement, causing extreme emotional frustration and insecurity.

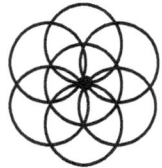

Can you bring these measurements into balance?

Yes, it is possible to bring these two measurements into balance. You simply must practice a spiritual discipline with great desire and consistency. Take note that the following chapters offer an excellent method of bringing these two measurements into balance in as little as one year.

Just keep reading. . .there is a lot more to cover!

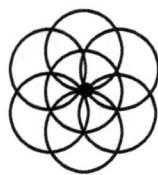

". . .so would the Holy Spirit release your vision and let you see the Great Rays shining from them, so unlimited that they reach to God. It is this shift to vision that is accomplished. . . .where the Great Rays replace the body in awareness."
A Course in Miracles

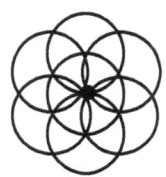

Portals of Power

Your Seven Sacred Chakras

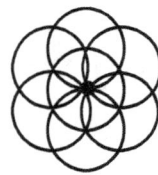

Your electromagnetic field

The rumbling of titanic boulders rolls across the sky. Suddenly the explosive bang of thunder shakes the very ground. Spear points of lightning bolts jab the earth and the animal kingdom cowers in caves and burrow for protection. They recognize the power of nature, its creative and destructive energy, and they respect and honor its presence, but do you?

Sure, you may come in from the rain and stay away from tall trees during a thunderstorm, but do you recognize, respect and honor the creative and destructive energy that sizzles from your very fingertips, from your mind?

You and every thing in this Universe emit electromagnetic currents. The stars and planets bombard the earth with shifting force fields and astrology tracks this phenomena with its calculations. As the wind and rain and drought mold the surface of the land, the air is also molded and enlivened by negative and positive ions. Animals migrate from plain to valley and stir the energy fields into small eddies and vortices. . .

. . .And every time you walk into a room you change the whole electromagnetic energy field by your simple presence.

Your mind is a mighty gyro spinning smoothly and creatively or spiraling in out-of-sinc rhythms of destruction. Your mental health is the barometer by which you can determine how creatively or destructively you are affecting yourself, others and the Universe. You are the only one who can bring your energy field back into balance.

Your aura is the complex spiraling electromagnetic field that spills over from your metabody, through your chakras, into your physical body and the world. As you learn to open your mind to peace it will direct the flow of energy through your Portals of Power into a controlled, harmonious and healing woven pattern.

This is your power, and this is your responsibility.

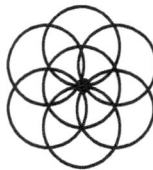

Your Root Portal of Power

The ever rising and descending force of life pulsates through this first power plant located at the base of the spine near the reproductive organs. This Portal of Power, like all other Portals, is constantly charged with energy for this is a window to your Soul. Through this window radiates Divine Love, Life Itself. As each Entity learns through its many lifetimes the basic lesson of survival, this Root Portal becomes more powerfully accessed. This Portal represents Life and Its desire to reproduce. At its lowest level of use sex is the focus. At its highest use, love unfolds.

The Sacred Word - Divinity

Divinity is your Soul's "DNA". You are created out of Divinity. So is everything around you. Without accepting, understanding and applying this truth into your world you will remain emotionally incomplete and depressed. Your Divinity was a gift given to you before your innumerable physical births. You can cleanse this first Portal of Power and make available to yourself the Divinity that is your rightful inheritance and once more be empowered to express the purity of creation, the spiritual love for others, for yourself, and for God.

The Sacred Color of Love - Radiant Red

The color of the most beautiful rose signifies love at its most romantic purity. Untouched by jealousy or lust, this color represents your highest expression of spiritual passion for your fellow man. The gift of deep appreciation, eternal faith and the purist of motives is offered by the Radiant Red that pours through this Portal.

The womb. The essence of gentle enfoldment and protection. The quiet peace of total contentment. The Love of God. Love flows through your Root Portal of Power as a deep rose tinted haze. Though this mist is not seen with the physical eyes, it can be felt and enjoyed by everyone. The true color of any Portal is not within the visible spectrum. The red that is associated with the Portal of Power is actually many octaves lower that the actual astral vibration. Red, however, becomes the visible symbol of Love and its waves of gentle giving that come from God, through you, to your world. As you work to cleanse and open your Root Portal of Power the rose tinted mist of God's Love will flow continuously, comforting you and those who are sent to you for comfort.

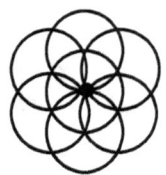

*Through this Portal the following issues
can be discovered and then healed.*

Death and Endings

This area includes:

1. Handling grief
2. Letting go of the old
3. Being willing to stop outgrown habits and discard the inappropriate.

Sexual Identity

This area includes:

1. Getting in touch with your masculine and feminine aspects ☯
2. Learning about your own sexual needs
3. Dealing successfully and satisfyingly with your sexual partner

(Note: not having a sexual partner does not affect the healing of this Portal.)

As you work on opening and cleansing this Portal of Power, these particular issues will begin to surface into your life in very concrete form in both your relationships and your physical body. Your personal scenario, however, will be uniquely your own. How clearly you will be able to recognize these issues will depend on how much into balance you have brought your Level of Soul Evolvement with your Level of Actualization. The more balanced these levels the greater the clarity you will have coupled with greater focused power.

By working on opening this Portal you will begin the process of bringing issues to the surface and finding the answers. Your whole life will be a spiraling journey along which the stages of denial, practice and accomplishment will occur and reoccur repeatedly.

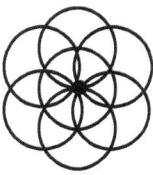

General Exercise and Journal Work

*Suggested Exercise to practice consistently
so that it becomes a habit and second nature*

1. What is your personal goal for the Portal of Power?

2. Make a list of those areas of your life that depress you, make you unhappy, cause to feel angry, and make you want to run away.

After each one say to yourself:
> "When I look at the world this way, I cannot see my own Divinity."

And then then say out loud:
> "I choose now to open to my Divine Self!"

3. Write on several 3x5 cards the following statement and carry one with you, tape one to the bathroom mirror, place one one your desk where you can see it,etc.

> "I choose now to open to my Divine Self!"

!And remember to look at it often!

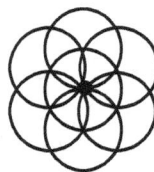

The Power of the Universe

You are most familiar with your physical body and generally how it functions. The spinal column is the main highway on which the signals from the brain pass to all parts of your body guiding them to perform in a balanced and healthy fashion. However, you may have not been aware of the subtle body that resides on the next level of existence. This subtle body, or metabody superimposes itself onto and into your physical body. This metabody also has a major channel, similar to the spinal column. On this channel are found the windows to your Soul, your Portals of Power, also called your chakras in Sanskrit. It is along this channel that the Power of the Universe dances and spirals like a Sacred Serpent as it shines through each window creating your radiant aura. Within this channel is also stored all your emotional memories from all your many lifetimes. Through each Portal of Power the Sacred Serpent's wisdom can be accessed and used to correct or enhance these memories.

The Sacred Serpent may rest patiently waiting for lifetimes, but once aroused She raises her head and commences her dance. At each window to your Soul She gazes outward flicking Her tongue with interest and excitement. Like flames the bright heat of Her rapidly moving tongue radiates through the Soul's windows, your chakras, exciting, energizing and empowering you and the world She touches. She is the Power of the Universe that spirals within you. She is the Holy Spirit. She is Life.

Since the most ancient of times the Eastern tradition has seen this energy flow as a serpent, and She is yours to follow and command!

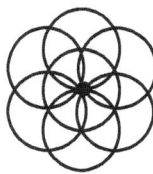

Your Navel Portal of Power

Physical strength and the power to literally move mountains comes from this window to the Soul. As a Pilgrim progresses through his many lifetimes learning about the physical world, he also learns how to actively utilize this Portal. From here life flows forth molding the universe. Physical strength is simply the end product of the power field emitted from the Navel Portal located near the intestines and surrounding organs. At its lowest level of use physical endurance is the result. At its highest come the ideas that mold and construct cities, highways and change the surface of the planet itself.

The Sacred Word - Balance

Located beneath your navel yet found on the channel that runs along your metabody is your Navel Portal of Power, the second window to your Soul. Here the balancing of your life and energies take place, and here you begin to funnel the power of God through you and into your world. Finding stability in an ever-changing world and discovering the stamina and energy to do the things necessary will be your focus as you open this Portal.

Teetering on the edge of life itself imbalance seems to be a constant factor needing consistent correction. You spend too much time, or too little time on what is asked of you. You have too much drive, or too little interest in your daily activities. You over commit, or run away. Now is the time to find balance in your life.

The Sacred Color of Power - Radiant Orange

Awake and hear the call of your ultimate purpose and function! The color of power, ambition and purpose is found in Radiant Orange. Energy sings through your being and lifts your spirits and the spirits of those around you through the strength and clarity this color brings.

Sunrise, sunset. The blazing glory of the orange flamed powerplant of theheaven the sun heats the world and the world lives. Within you is also a flaming orange powerplant. It rests waiting to blaze forth through your second Portal of Power bringing you the energy and the force necessary to express life powerfully. As you open this Portal you invite the Sacred Serpent to flick Her flaming tongue through this second window to the Soul, and the orange glow of sunrise and sunset will bring power to your body, your relationships and your mind.

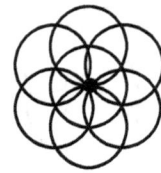

*Through this Portal the following issues
can be discovered and then healed.*

Finding Balance in Your Diet

The food you eat replenishes and sustains your physical health. Thus, this tool which carries you to wherever you must be to express your function in this life, must be respected and maintained. Choosing foods incorrectly shows a lack of interest and responsibility toward yourself. Choosing correctly brings a sense of satisfaction and well- being.

Finding Balance in Your Physical Activities

Moving your body stimulates circulations, strengthens muscles, enhances your immune system, releases emotional tension, and much more. Exercising too little shows a lack of enthusiasm for life. Exercising too much is a form of obsession and comes from fear, not joy. Learning to move your body according to its needs brings relaxation.

Finding Balance in Your Thoughts

Your mind needs both stimulation and rest. Your mind needs to learn and also to teach. Your mind needs to express creativity, as well as appropriate fantasy. Your mind needs a good night's rest. Recognizing an over or under worked mind is easy - thoughts become chaotic and confusing. Learning to use your mind in all its many possibilities brings clarity and insight.

As you work on the issues attached to the Navel Portal of Power you will often find golden opportunities presenting themselves for you to apply what you must learn. Time and energy demands will fluctuate uncomfortably and it will be up to you to recognize your needs and design a balanced lifestyle for yourself. No one can do this for you. You can read and study and listen to advisors, but the ultimate decision of what will be correct for balance in your life, is yours!

Now that we have looked more closely at what these issues can be, you can continue on your pathway of healing by practicing the following exercise consistently. This will create a healthy habit of balance for your life.

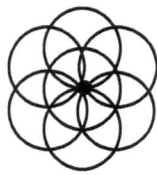

General Exercise and Journal Work
Suggested Exercise to practice consistently
so that it becomes a habit and second nature

1. What is your personal goal for the Portal of Power?

2. Under each heading list the improvement you **can and will do for yourself** to bring balance in your life **over the next week.** Remember to be specific and choose only what you can succeed in. By doing this consistently you will form a solid habit of monitoring your own health and well being.

DIET:

EXERCISE:

SLEEP:

WORKTIME:

PLAYTIME:

You may want to stick this to your refrigerator
and review it each morning and update it each week.

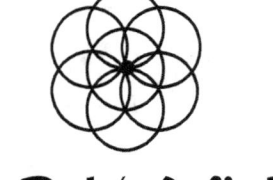

The Body's Windows

Seven major Portals of Power can be found within your body. These Portals of Power are windows to the great expanse of Divinity from which you were created. After the Cycle of Alpha to Omega began, the expression of Divine Life seemed to focus itself down and become more and more limited. When this devolution reached its lowest point, the most concrete form of life, man, found himself encapsulated. His body became his prison. Yet, even here Divinity could not be fully blocked. Your Portals of Power demonstrate this.

These seven Portals reside near groupings of major organs and glands. This is not accidental. The organs and glands gain the energy to pump and flow and process because of the power radiating from these Portals. It is your Divinity which gives you life, your Divinity that is this power source. Each Portal of Power pulsates at its own vibrational frequency. This is sometimes seen by sensitives and individuals and is what causes the aura which surrounds your body.

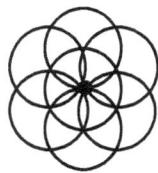

Your Solar Plexus Portal of Power

From the Solar Plexus Portal of Power a glimpse into the wisdom of God can be gained. Therefore, from this window comes the understanding which is sought and then found as the Soul progresses through the level of Aspirant. To what is this Soul aspiring? Here the Soul draws upon the power plant that can answer the following questions: "What is my purpose in life and how can I begin to express it?" The mind is reaching for understanding and through this window is glimpsed the answer. At the lowest level of use mind over analyzes, but at its highest the successful teacher of God is born.

The Sacred Word – Integration

At a point just below the ribcage is found the third window to your Soul. Through this window you will discover how to bring the aspects of body, mind and spirit into an integrated framework of expression. Life and understanding will fill your mind and build clear powers of observation. Through this Portal real integration and understanding can be found.

You are the light, yet you experience yourself through the prism of belief in worldly form. The more focused you are on the details of your life, the more fragmented you seem to be. Life becomes a jumble of experiences, disconnected to each other. Decisions become random, discipline inconsistent, and thinking chaotic. As you open this Portal the power to bring all aspects of your life into an integrated design will surge through you into the world. As you work on integrating aspects of your body, your relationships and your mind, your identity as a spiritual whole will strengthen.

The Sacred Color of Understanding - Radiant Yellow

Light pours into your mind, opening a channel of understanding and expression. The color of the sun brings intellectual clarity. Yellow floods your thinking with brilliance and radiates a mental state of earthly wisdom. Yellow once more expresses the highest level of the worship of the sun, the intellect of man.

Understanding brings the whole picture, the overview, the coalescing of a kaleidoscope of experiences into one point. Just as a confusing array of colored tiles blends visually into a mosaic of structure and purpose, so too will the confusing input of information and insight blend into one point of personal structure and purpose. Through this third window to the Soul the golden glow of understanding brightens a mind dulled by confusion. Sunlight shines brilliant clarity into the deepest recesses of your thinking and all becomes illuminated. You understand!

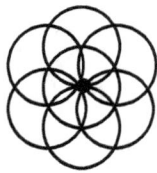

*Through this Portal the following issues
can be discovered and then healed.*

Integrating Body, Mind and Spirit

You are a spiritual being. Your Portals of Power are the doors through which the power, love and wisdom of your spirituality can flow into your body and then express outward into your world. As you work to open and cleanse your Solar Plexus Portal of Power you are allowing all aspects of yourself and your world to be brought together as an integrated whole. You begin to see clearer and stronger connections between cause and effect. The need to appreciate that you are a complex unit interacting with a world that is an extension of your complex but unified self will grow. You no longer experience your thoughts as random and out of control. Instead, you begin to see the source of all your ideas as either coming from fear and defensiveness, or from love. You begin to see yourself as responsible for yourself and the world you inhabit.

Understanding and Decision making

Through this third Portal to your Soul comes the understanding that will guide all your decisions. Without clear understanding, decision making becomes chaotic and/or impossible. As you gain an integrated view of cause and effect, as well as your role and responsibility in your personal life and the world around you, you will be able to make the correct decision that will guide your actions. Clear thinking brings decisiveness.

As you open and cleanse your Solar Plexus Portal of Power you will find yourself gaining the ability to view yourself and others clearly. From this clarity will come the strength to move forward and be truly helpful.

Once more I celebrate the progress you are making and remind you that levels of lessons occur in a spiraling movement. Therefore, your work will continue as as you learn and accomplish and then face higher levels of challenges. Remember, however, that you take with you the strength, experience and insight you have already gained

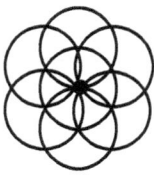

General Exercise and Journal Work
*Suggested Exercise to practice consistently
so that it becomes a habit and second nature*

1. What is your personal goal for the Portal of Power?

2. In one sentence identify one recent and/or on-going challenge you must face:

3. List the lessons you can learn from this challenge:

4. List the people who are and will be touched by these lessons:

5. List the rewards you can gain from succeeding with this challenge:

Notice how your personal challenge affects so many in so many ways!

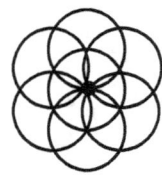

The Earth's Windows

The planet Earth is also a body and it, too, has Portals of Power, windows to Heaven. There are certain places, towns, mountains and valleys that serve this purpose. These spots on the planet are vortices that create an inflow and outflow of energy giving forth life and balancing the electromagnetic fields. Many of the world's cathedrals, Indian mounds and ancient stone rings are found at these spots. From the most ancient of times man has felt these power sources and has reverently paid homage. Pilgrimages are made to these areas since they call to individuals to once more align their energy fields with those of the planet. At these places a celebration of life occurs with all the kingdoms - mineral, plant, animal, human and spiritual - participating in harmony.

Parallel Kingdoms

The Kingdoms of Life divide into five.
Each Kingdom evolves and grows and divines
Its purpose and function,
Its pathway to God.

The Mineral Kingdom offers a bedrock of FAITH.

The Plant Kingdom offers SUSTENANCE and STRENGTH.

The Animal Kingdom offers AMBASSADORS of Friendship.

The Human Kingdom offers CHALLENGES and LESSONS.

The Spiritual Kingdom offers the GUIDANCE that leads
each Kingdom to safety and the peace that will heal.

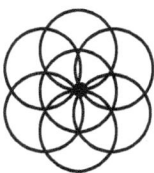

Your Heart Portal of Power

The heart is the seat of mercy and forgiveness. Through this window shines the love of the Christ energy. From this Portal of Power comes the forgiveness that heals the Soul and then the world. As a Probationary Disciple the Soul has made a commitment to spiritual growth. This Portal becomes the power plant that sustains this desire and gives meaning to its outer expression. Through the use of this Portal the Soul can begin true healing - the healing of the mind of guilt, fear and anger. At the lowest point of use its power is focused into forming organizations to change the world. At its highest use of power the Soul changes and the world cannot help but follow.

The Sacred Word - Health

Centered within your metabody on the channel that feeds your Soul is the Heart Portal of Power. Through this window are discovered those areas of your mind closed to wholeness and change. Through this window you can invite the Sacred Serpent to help heal your broken heart. As you work on this Portal you will be addressing those areas within you needing forgiveness. This will lead to a natural healing in your body, your mind and your world. You will begin by looking at the true meaning of health and how this leads directly to rebirth. No one can continue on his Soul's journey to transcendence unless he allows himself to be healed and reborn. You start now.

Health equals wholeness. Wholeness is the removal of all barriers and the restoration of a splintered and darkened mind. Health then will be the opening of your mind to all issues that would block wholeness. The acceptance of Wisdom will help you to forgive the wrongs of others as well as yourself. Through this forgiveness the walls of guilt, fear and anger will tumble down. The gentle expanse of a peaceful and healed mind will remain.

The Sacred Color of Rebirth - Radiant Green

Spring: the sprouting of buds, leaves shooting forth fresh and new from branches that have rested through the calm of winter. Rebirth once more occurs and green becomes the color of newness, healing and life. Green offers another beginning where the old has died, and life once again, fresh and vibrant explodes forth showering your world with hope.

The gentle healing shimmer of green floats like a clouds through your Heart Portal. The lightest green of the newly sprouting leaves to the deepest forest green of the everliving pine flows in waves from your Heart Portal as you allow your life to evolve and for you to be reborn. Holding rigidly to thoughts, ideas, opinions and emotions will only block this window to your Soul. The willingness to evolve and adapt will open this Portal so that you can begin your new life.

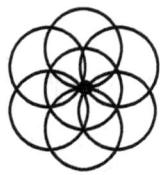

Through this Portal the following issues
can be discovered and then healed.

Lowering the Walls of Guilt, Fear and Anger

Health, a main aspect of the issues attached to the Heart Portal of Power, refers to the wholeness that occurs when you feel one with everyone and everything. The main stumbling block to health, therefore, will be the walls you place between you and others, between you and the world, between you and God and between you and yourself! The building blocks which form the foundation of this wall are the emotions of guilt, fear and anger. Many believe that they experience only one of these emotions at any time and are free from the others. Not so! When you feel unworthy (guilt) you fear rejection (fear of punishment) and attempt to redirect the punishment by proving another's guilt (this coping technique is called anger). Thus the Deadly Cycle of all three emotions is in play. By recognizing the full dynamic at work in yourself, you begin the process of lowering your walls and becoming whole once more.

Forgiving Yourself and Others

Are you willing to let go of your judgments about others, the world and yourself? Until you are, you will keep the ramparts around yourself high and strong, removing yourself from healing However, when you are ready to say to yourself, "Maybe I am wrong, and there is another way of seeing this," then the process of forgiveness can begin. Forgiveness brings a release from pain and does not include self-punishment as an attempt at correction. When you can humbly remove your stubborn desire to see wrong in others, you will be surprised at how quickly your mind will be filled with a compassion that is both powerful and healing.

As you open and cleanse the Heart Portal of Power you are asking to be shown those areas of your life where you have been too stubborn to release judgments. Now is the time when you can continue to allow real healing to be expressed in and through you by your willingness to be shown anew with open heart and mind.

Love blesses the progress you are making and the gift of appreciation you give yourself and the world as you lower the barriers to guilt, fear and anger and replace them with the Healing Cycle of innocence, safety and forgiveness.

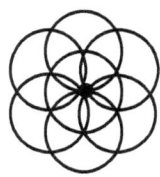

General Exercise and Journal Work
Suggested Exercise to practice consistently
so that it becomes a habit and second nature

1. What is your personal goal for the Portal of Power?

2. List 6 people who have *hurt you* in the past or present and list next to each name what they did to hurt you (ex. abandoned you, abused you, invalidated you,etc.) and then stretch yourself spiritually and list why they needed to do this to you.
(ex. self-protection, trying to help, training, etc.)

Names	what he/she did	why you think they did this
1.		
2.		
3.		
4.		
5.		
6.		

3. Now list 6 people who *you have hurt* in the past or present and list next to each name what you did to hurt them, and then why you felt you needed to act this way.

Names	what you did	why you think you did this
1.		
2.		
3.		
4.		
5.		
6.		

Now contemplate the results . . .Interesting, isn't it?

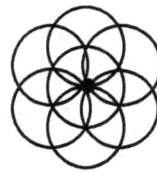

The Celestial Radiance

Each of your seven personal Portals of Power radiates an interlocking network of pathways forming a pulsating, flowing field of energy. These central power plants create a winding surge of Life that rises, descends and spirals upward once more through and around you. This pulsating life force energizes the organs and glands surrounding the power plants and sends extending tendrils of energy through the rest of the network. Every cell of your body feels this excitement. Each power plant or Portal glows with the Radiance of Life and sends a specific and important signal from Divinity to you and the world.

The Celestial Radiance gives the promise of eternal peace. Your personal and radiant aura offers your message of peace and love to the world. It surrounds you, caresses you and gently or powerfully touches the people in your life. Your personal radiance is both intimate and worldly. It flows from your Portals of Power as a harmonic weaving of rainbow light higher in "octave" than the eye can see, but always felt by the heart.

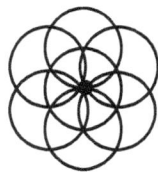

Your Throat Portal of Power

The window to the true Disciple's role lies within and around the throat. This is the Portal of listening, expressing, and leadership. From this Portal comes the ability to share the innovative teachings of eternal truth. Great power can be channeled through this window. However, a Soul must progress sufficiently in desire and understanding. Trying to utilize this Portal unprepared will cause "burn out". Yes, it is possible to use the power flowing through a Portal without having fully been prepared for its secrets. Nevertheless, when one attempts to channel the power radiating through this window onto the international level of service possible, his motives must be aligned correctly and his body, the vehicle of expression strong enough for the task. At its lowest level of use the Throat Portal can offer world renowned oratory, books and art. At the highest level the world's great spiritual teachings are created.

The Sacred Word - Communication

Through this fifth window to the Soul flows forth the power and inspiration to be a leader. Leadership includes more than instruction for others. Leadership is the ability to listen and then to guide; to be willing to help then offer appropriate assistance. Leadership is a natural power that can only occur when others feel true respect for you and your judgment. To reach out and experience a sense of oneness with another, to understand what he wishes to share with you, and to clearly and appropriately share with him: This is communication. Only a person willing to open to another with a sincere interest in another's life can offer true communication. Only a person willing to keep no secrets, but to be open with his heart's desires can truly share. Communication includes the willingness to listen without the need to add to or subtract from another's ideas. Appropriate communication includes the willingness to offer one's own thoughts clearly and gently.

The Sacred Color of Service - Radiant Bright Blue

Being of service to others brings no loss at all, but instead rewards you with fulfillment. The color of bright blue represents the greatest gift you can give to another, yourself. Clear blue enfolds both you and another in a womb of gentle and flowing communication. Clear blue protects, comforts and connects you and your world, one with the other. To serve is your only true profession. Service is the way to help others, and by helping others you are helping yourself for you find real satisfaction. True service, however, means that you are truly of help. Too often help is seen as correcting the mistakes of others. This only hinders another's progress. Real help is supporting another's spiritual journey by demonstrating your own progress. Start to shine your own bright blue light of helpfulness now.

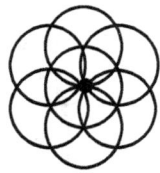

*Through this Portal the following issues
can be discovered and then healed.*

Listening Truly

The three relationship Portals of Power are the Solar Plexus, the Heart and the Throat. By opening all three so that they work in unison, real communication can occur. As you have learned, opening your Solar Plexus Portal allows you to see situations as an integrated whole. As you open your Heart Portal greater perspective gives you the courage to allow your walls and barriers to drop and forgiveness of yourself and others naturally follows.

Now, as you practice to open your Throat Portal of Power you will be able to build on this broadened perspective and forgiving heart to guide your ability to truly hear. The deepest need, hidden by emotional duress will now be heard by you. The most hesitant offer of help and assistance will also now be heard. The first evokes the response of compassion, the second gratitude.

Appropriate Responses

No matter what anyone says or does there are only two possible messages underlying what is being offered. Either one is extending love and support in the only way one knows how, or one is calling desperately for help and support in the only way one knows how.

Each of these messages when heard clearly for what it is will elicit from you the only appropriate response - your own message of love, support and gratitude. Here, clear and honest communication finally occurs and with it will come the specific inspiration for what to say and what to do.

As you work on all three of these Portals of Power you will discover an acceleration of opportunities to use your growing understanding, forgiveness and communication skills. Be proud of what you are accomplishing and know that the Power of the Universe needs you for the healing of the world.

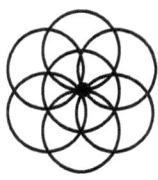

General Exercise and Journal Work
Suggested Exercise to practice consistently
so that it becomes a habit and second nature

1. What is your personal goal for the Portal of Power?

There are only two messages that any individual is sending forth:

     A - Help - The person is extending help in the only way he/she know how
     B - Fear - The person is calling for help in the only way he/she knows how

Keep track of any challenging conversations and interactions you have with anyone over the next seven weeks. List each one and make note of the messages coming from you and others.

Conversation Theme :	The other person: fear or help?	My message: fear or help?
1.		
2.		
3.		
4.		
5.		
6.		
7.		
8.		

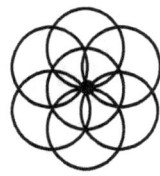

The Rhythm of Color

Color is movement, waves of energy that wash through you, over you and around your world. Each radiant aura color vibrates at a different speed. Each color gently feathers your mind and body, or vigorously massages them. From earthly to spiritual, from Root Portal to Crown Portal, your radiant aura colors proceed shining through each Portal of Power filling your aura with a celestial symphony of vibration unheard by the ear.

White is the most spiritual of colors. When added to any other color, white serves as a softening agent to add purity and comfort to the vibration. Just as you might turn the sound down on a radio, yet still retain the musical notes, white quiets your radiant aura, gentling its message. Celestial pastels offer safety and peace.

Black is inverted energy. Black represents receptivity, a pulling in rather than a sending out, a possessiveness of spirit rather than a generosity. Black reverses the polarity of your aura by blocking your Portals of Power. When this occurs the vibration of black will seem to muddy the radiant aura colors. This is why the visible color of black is often experienced as an emotionally depressing color.

You will "feel" these colors radiating from other individuals, and may occasionally "see" them. When this happens you have simply, yet importantly allowed your mind to open to a higher level of communication.

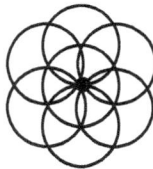

Your Forehead Portal of Power

Traditionally called the third eye this Portal of Power radiates the integration of worldly matters with spiritual insight. Thus, wisdom is born. Here the Soul begins to know. This is a level far beyond the intellectual understanding achieved through the Solar Plexus Portal of Power. This power plant radiates communication given to the Soul by the Spiritual Masters. At its lowest level of use altered consciousness lifts the veils between dimensions. At its highest level nirvana is seen and Heaven found.

The Sacred Word - Wisdom

As the tongue of the Sacred Serpent flickers and dances through this sixth window to the Soul brilliant flashes of wisdom fill your being with serenity. Through this Portal you can explore the inner levels of life, feel the flow of energy throughout your metabody, and travel the many astral planes of existence. Be prepared for an eventful time. Wisdom is an inner vision. Wisdom lets you see more than your simple physical sense shows you. Wisdom accesses Sacred understanding for you can see from above, below, between and beyond and through the many levels of existence. As you work on this Portal you will be inviting the Wisdom of the Universe to guide you. It will help you understand both your physical body and metabody, as well as your multi-dimensional relationships.

The Sacred Color of Serenity - Radiant Deep Blue

The night sky draws you deeply into the serene shelter of your mind. Here God resides and here you enter the Living Temple, the most holy of holies. Deep blue, the darkest and richest of blues brings forth the memory of your Divinity and reminds those who touch your world, of theirs. Peace - deep, profound and undisturbed - cloaks you as you allow radiant deep blue to fill the recesses of your being.

This comforting blanket of love gently weaves its calming effect around your mind. Serenity comes from knowing. For when you know you can then do what will be the obvious and the best. Here the maternal gentleness of the Sacred Serpent can be found. She waits patiently to offer you this gift. Delay no longer. It is time to fill your body, your relationships and your mind with the love of the Divine Mother.

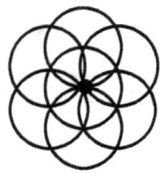

*Through this Portal the following issues
can be discovered and then healed.*

<u>Tapping into the Mystical</u>

Through your Forehead Portal of Power you receive the mystical experiences that confirm your own Divinity and show you the karmic threads which bind you to everyone around you. Although this Portal is called the third "eye", most people erroneously associate it with simple psychic power. However, the ability to know who is on the phone before you answer it, for example, is a less elevated process and actually comes through your Solar Plexus Portal of Power. Through your Forehead Portal comes the mystical experiences that bring you visions of heavenly grandeur!

To open and cleanse this Portal means that you must learn how to meditate and begin reaching for the inner Silence, that space in your mind where thought stops and insight is given. Let us look more closely at this issue and how you can enhance your own ability to meditate.

Life is a flow of experiences. Life begins with the knowledge of God, for this joint Identity is Who We are. Somewhere, somehow you have blocked that full knowledge and seem to walk through emotionally fragmented experiences. Time and space form the organizational files for these fragments. The world now reflects your random and often emotionally disturbing files. As you begin to focus away from the fragments and inward to the center of your mind, you fly through a seeming hurricane into the eye where it is calm.

By visually focusing on the Sacred Symbols each day you are automatically focusing your mind into its calm center. Each Symbol becomes a non-verbal prayer. Each of the powerful, yet deceptively simple prayers unlocks the inner door to the Wisdom of the Universe offering the specific guidance you need. These Symbols, their colors, power words and prayers combine to strengthen your resolve, balance your energies and bring your mind peace.

Are there other forms of mediation? Of course! Use those that call to you and bring you success. But remember, you must do it! To gain the vision of Heaven you must learn how to see It. Meditation is the way. . .

. . .and may your Soul's progress be swift!

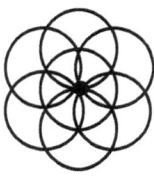

General Exercise and Journal Work
Suggested Exercise to practice consistently
so that it becomes a habit and second nature

1. What is your personal goal for the Portal of Power?

2. What is your present meditation schedule:

3. What kinds of meditation practices have you tried and which ones have been the most comfortable and successful:

4. Create a new and improved daily, weekly and monthly meditation schedule:

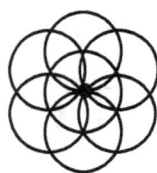

Be gentle and patient with yourself. . .

You have waited thousands of years preparing for just this acceleration. As your Portals of Power begin to reveal your hidden emotional memories you may feel as if you have stepped onto a mental roller coaster ride. Learn to relax and know you are not alone. The Masters of the Universe, the Angels of Heaven and your Spiritual Helpers are with you. These Spiritual Helpers will guide you through your accelerated progress. Remember, also, that helpers and teachers here on the physical plane can be found to ease your fears and discomfort. You are not alone.

By following this home study course you may open psychic experiences for yourself. When they are comfortable for you encourage them. Should anything become definitely uncomfortable and emotionally disturbing, STOP. Never do anything in your life that does not lead to comfort. The next step is to ask in meditation for insight into your experience. This can bring you understanding and comfort Usually a little insight will be all that is necessary to ease your mind and help you continue on your accelerated journey.

Remember, you cannot hurt yourself, others or do anything wrong with the Sacred Symbols and this home study course. Your willingness with a little discipline is all that is needed to enhance the healing power within. The sacred energy of life is stirring within you at this very moment. It is eternally ready to dance within your Soul. Simply work with this course and It will do the rest. This is all It desires.

Do not deny It. . .for It is You.!

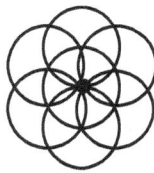

Your Crown Portal of Power

At physical birth this window is still open and symbolically closes down as the baby's skull completes its growth. For the rest of a Soul's life, and through its many evolving lives, the goal is to wash clear, window by window, Portal by Portal the haze which keeps the Soul from knowing its own Divinity. No one can use this Portal of Power fully unless his Soul is truly ready. Alpha to Omega is both a point of clarity and the journey to it. When the Soul has completed all that is necessary to end its karma this final Portal opens fully. Now Heaven becomes a constant reality. The veils that hide Life dissolve. All Portals of Power are clear and luminous. A Master is born!

The Sacred Word - Revelation

Here you have come to the final window to your Soul. Through this Portal a newborn child's spirit focuses inward and downward thrusting life into the newly formed physical body. This life rushes down the subtle channel and waits patiently beneath the Root Portal. Not until the maturing individual asks with great sincerity, "What is life" will the Serpent begin her dance! You have asked this question. The Sacred Serpent has begun to dance and now with this Portal it is time for Spirit to be revealed. The Light of Heaven shines through his Portal and you can feel the rush of life, see the radiance of love, feel the movement of creation. Through this window is God. Throughout time masters have walked the earth teaching many methods of how to access this experience. The path is simple, yet profound. The Sacred Symbols will lead you Home.

The Sacred Color of Spirit - Radiant Violet

The Kingdom has come! Your royalty is unquestioned. Your reign benign and eternal. Violet floods your kingdom knighting all aspects of the world, commanding respect from the four directions, uniting earth and Heaven. Violet is the color of your royal robe, the symbol of Divine rank. You are a child of God, fully expressing your spirituality. Your royal vestment pours forth as a gently woven cloud of violet and purple from your Crown Portal of Power. This raiment flows and swirls around your form infusing it with the essence of your reality. This is Spirit.

Spirit is the manifestation of God's Mind. This is God's Child. This is you.

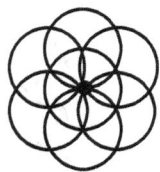

Through this Portal the following issues
can be discovered and then healed.

The Zen master sits for hours on end, year after year, reaching for the state of bliss that can be attained through this Portal. You, too, have been reaching for this transcendent experience, but, like the Zen master you can merely invite this gift. To be given it is up to the Universe Itself when It knows you will be ready.

Through this Portal is sent the Light of Life Which rushes down your inner channel to rest below the Root Portal. This energy shines upward bringing radiance to all seven Portals. It is up to you, however, to open and cleanse each window to your Soul to allow the full brilliance of the Serpent's light to shine through you. The final window to be rinsed clear is always the Crown Portal. For only the most sincere and consistently dedicated will be able to reach this high. Through your efforts you have brought greater clarity even to this most sacred window.

Is your work finished? Will you have reached the level of Zen master with bliss your constant state of mind at the end of this Program? Probably not. This does not mean failure. On the contrary, you will work hard and attain another and much more advanced level of personal growth. You will spiral successfully through many and varied challenges. You will graduate to the next level. I celebrate your progress!

What must you do as you complete this journey? Why the same that you have always needed to do - enjoy life, bring willingness and forgiveness to everything you do and continue to ask for God's Will. You will be guided to those tools that can help you spiral successfully through the next level of life experiences. Perhaps you may choose to go continue to use the Sacred Symbols as a focusing tool for an extended period of time. This will surely help. As you stretch and grow you touch the world with hope and it offers its thanks.

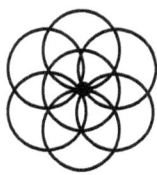

General Exercise and Journal Work
Suggested Exercise to practice consistently
so that it becomes a habit and second nature

1. What is your personal goal for the Portal of Power?

2. Who or what do you believe God to be?

3. What do you believe is your relationship to God?

4. What do you believe is the purpose God has given you?

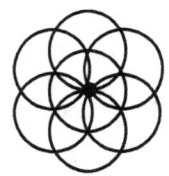

The Seven Great Rays

*The Seven Great Rays entwine to ignite
the one central fire of life.
And you are each given a torch to carry forth
into the darkness of the world
to lead the frightened and lost to safety.*

*The Seven Sacred Symbols represent
the seven elemental concepts that ignite the Universe.
You are mandated to guard, teach, and offer
these Sacred Symbols to
all who are sent to you.*

*Do not deny this responsibility!
For only you can help those bonded to you
through karmic law.*

You are the guardians of the flames!

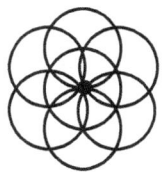

The Sacred Symbols

*How to Open, Balance and Empower
Your Seven Portals of Power*

and

Accelerate Your Soul's Progress

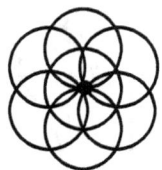

"God's teachers have God's Word behind their symbols. . .
Raising them from. . . symbols to the Call of Heaven itself.

A Course in Miracles

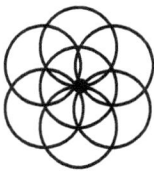

The power of the Word...

"No peace is possible until His Word is heard around the world..."
A Course in Miracles

Yantras
The MostAncient of Tools

You have probably heard of the term *mantra*, a Sanskrit word for a divine sound that is repeated in order to deepen the experience of meditation. The most well known mantra is the Sacred Sound *"OM"*. Few, however, have heard of the term *yantra*, which is a powerful geometric form drawn to represent Sacred Sounds and used in worship.

"OM" is the primordial and subtle vibration of the Universe. It is from the vibration of this Sacred Word that all sound comes, and all matter manifests. The *yantra* for the Sacred Sound *"OM"* is drawn as a perfect circle.

There is a device called a "tonoscope" which demonstrates very graphically how the power of Sacred Sound creates form. The tonoscope is a tube suspended over a thin membrane covered by a bed of chemical dust. When sounds are played and repeated above the tonoscope, designs form in the dust. And when *"OM"* is repeated at the proper pitch a perfect circle forms. Thus, when the perfect sound is uttered, out of the dust emerges the perfect form, a *yantra*.

Each of the Sacred Symbols are *yantras*, a powerful geometric forms. Each begins with the *yantra* for *"OM"*, the circle, and then geometrically expands into greater and greater complexity.

As you focus on the seven Sacred Symbols, the power of these yantras command the opening of each of your chakras, or Portals of Power inviting the primordial and divine energy of "OM", or the Holy Spirit, to flow up, out and through you. In this way you create and heal yourself and your world.

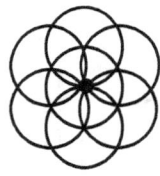

Sacred Geometry
Building the Sacred Symbols

The Greek philosopher, Pythagorus, studied both the Egyptian and Chaldean sciences, compared them to the Hindu and Hebrew philosophies and created a system of numbers that is the foundation of mathematics today. He saw numbers representing the rhythms of the Universe, both melody and building block. Geometry and music became metaphors for humanity and the tools for transcendent insight and personal growth.

Even before Pythagorus, those who used numbers were highly regarded in the ancient world as priests and shamans, or people of intense power. The architects and builders, musicians and poets were seen as holy men and women, and their sacred tools were closely guarded secrets. The placement of each stone, each building, each city needed to be exact and honored with the proper ritual and celebrations. The edifices were temples to the living God, the cities gathering places for those who would worship within.

From the circle geometric construction can produce the triangle, the square and a continuing extension of shapes. Here the rhythm of the Universe, God's Word, can be drawn, built and then seen in concrete form. The geometric patterns of all forms represent God's Word and thus we are surrounded by the symbols of His Love.

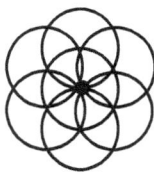

Using The Sacred Symbols

How to Open, Balance and Empower
Your Seven Portals of Power

Simply look at each of these seven Sacred Symbols in sequence for a minimum of 30 seconds to as much as two minutes for a total of 7 to 14 minutes each day.

These Symbols work for you, you do not work for them!

As you focus you immerse yourself in the power of sacred geometry, experience the holiness of the Word, and affirm your Divinity by aligning yourself with the Spiritual Hierarchy as you repeat the prayers.

Though deceptively simple, using these Sacred Symbols daily places you under the guidance of the Spiritual Hierarchy, and creates a clear channel of wisdom from your Inner Self to your functioning mind.

These Sacred Symbols enhance the powerful changes that take place within you as you use this very unique and exquisite gift sent from Heaven Itself to you. Your consistent discipline lifts you higher than the astral planes and gently places your mind in the company of the transcended Masters.

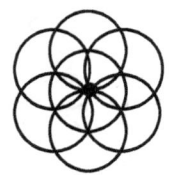

Divinity
The Key to your Root Portal of Power
in Radiant Red

(You may color in this symbol yourself)

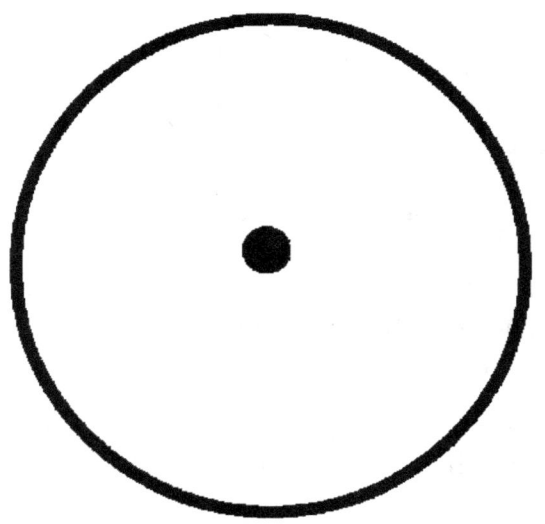

***"I open to my Divine Self,
and feel the love of God in me and around me!"***

Throughout time the mind of humanity has seen the Circle as representative of All That Is, the One. Drawn within this meditative tool you will find a focus point. As you look at this shape and this point your mind will meld with its archetypal meaning:

"Here is Oneness and I am within its center."

This first step up the geometric ladder can set the tone for all meditation. It forms the simplest of mandalas, the circular pictures used since ancient time to raise consciousness. To raise your consciousness simply focus on the center point, then allow your eye to roam around the perimeter, moving in a clockwise direction - the direction of the positive flow of universal energy.

The time you spend using this symbol is an invitation to remember your own Divinity.

72

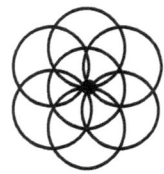

Balance
The Key to your Navel Portal of Power
in Radiant Orange
(You may color in this symbol yourself)

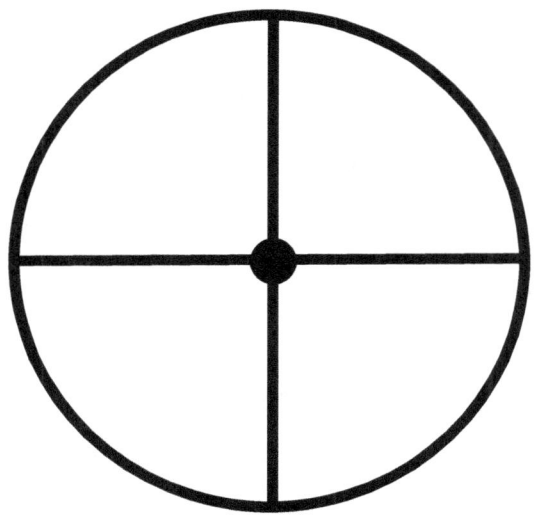

"All is in balance in my life.
I feel the flow of power through me."

The Power of God enters your conscious mind as you climb the next rung on the geometric ladder to transcendence. Here the horizontal line of the material plane is crossed by the vertical line of spirituality. At the place where the Power of God touches the world is the focus point, representing you. As you look at this central point your mind is filled with the balance necessary to perform on the material plane. Without the guidance of your Divine Self your life would become chaotic from imbalance. To gain this stability simply look at the central point and allow the Sacred Symbol for spirituality, and the balance this brings to enter your mind.

All you need do is focus.
Your willingness and discipline allows this symbol to work for you.

73

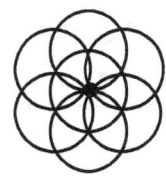

Integration

The Key to your Solar Plexus Portal of Power
in Radiant Yellow

(You may color in this symbol yourself)

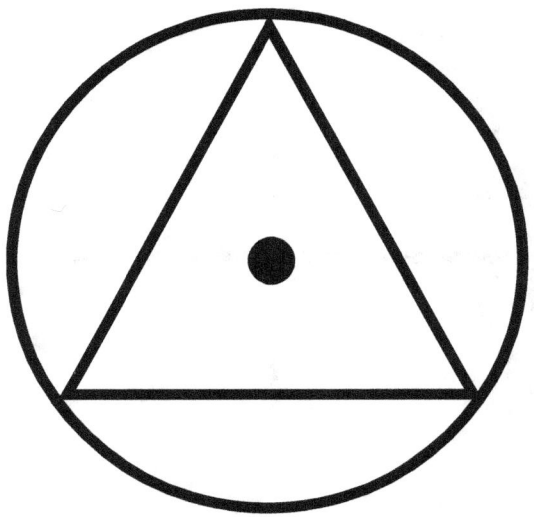

"I integrate and grow through my experience.
I am beginning to truly understand."

Through the use of the previous Sacred Symbols you have allowed Divine Guidance into your mind and therefore into your world. You have reached the next rung on the ladder. Here is the universal symbol for integration - the integration of body, mind and spirit. This meditative tool opens you to the full and balanced expression of life in all areas. From this experience comes the understanding that gives you the ability to make clear decisions.

To cleanse and empower your thinking process,
once more focus on the central point that represents you,
surrounded by the expression of the body, mind and spirit
that is contained within the Circle of God.

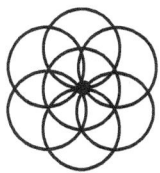

health

The Key to your heart Portal of Power
in Radiant Green

(You may color in this symbol yourself)

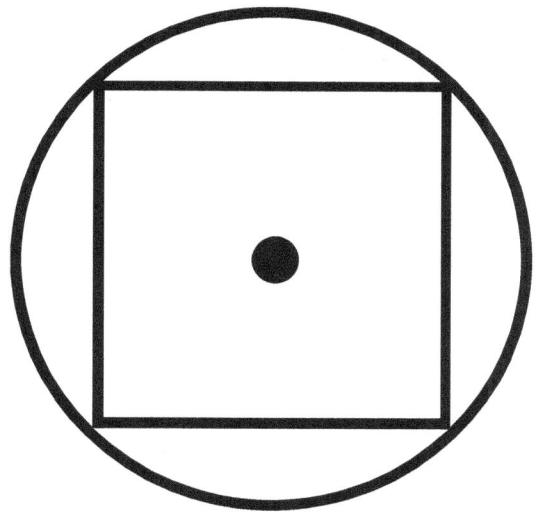

"My mind opens to wholeness and health.
I am being reborn each moment."

The integration of your life experiences and the clarity of decision-making that results from the use of the previous Sacred Symbol leads directly to the next shape, the Square, the next geometric rung. The four equally placed points of this shape build the foundation stone for a strong body - the vehicle of expression you must use on this plane of existence. As you focus on the central point of this Sacred Symbol you will find the opening of your heart. The walls of guilt, fear and anger separating you from others, from yourself, and from God, crumble.

The sense of wholeness that comes from this opening heals
your mind, your relationships, your body and your world.
Health is the result.

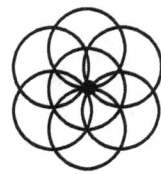

Communication
The Key to your Throat Portal of Power
in Radiant Clear Blue
(You may color in this symbol yourself)

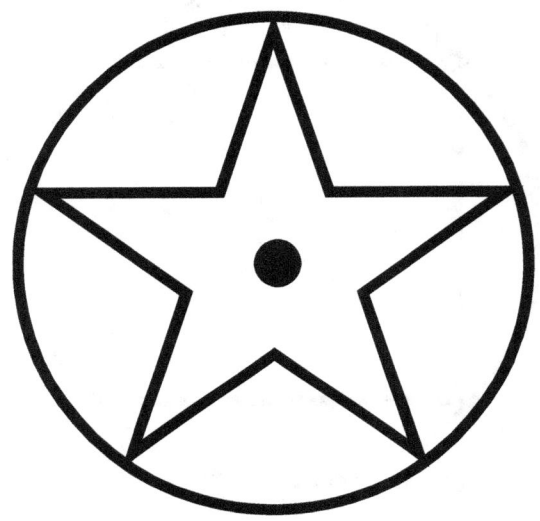

"I share and communicate love to all.
I am God's servant."

The stars in the heavens radiantly shine forth giving the message of God's eternal love. The five pointed star becomes the next geometric shape to carry you higher on your own journey to Heaven. To accomplish this you must reach out to others and help them understand and grow also. By focusing on this Sacred Symbol you offer yourself as a tool for teaching others, and you teach what you must learn for yourself! Communication of the glorious lesson of wholeness through the demonstration of your life is empowered by the use of this meditative tool.

You become the star by whose light
those who must follow can navigate.

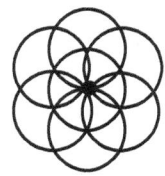

Wisdom
The Key to your Forehead Portal of Power
in Radiant Deep Blue
(You may color in this symbol yourself)

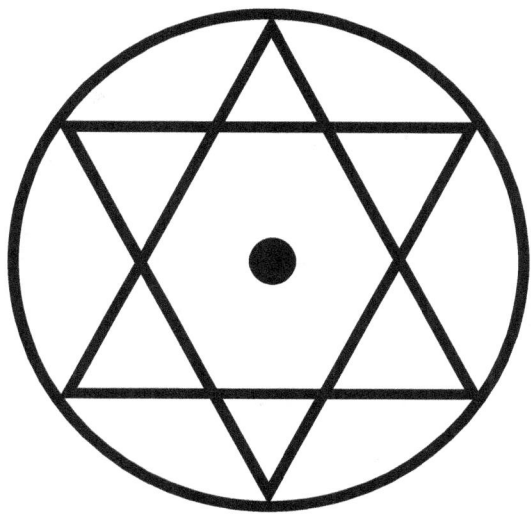

"Wisdom floods my mind and I know.
Serenity fills my days and nights."

The ancient symbol of wisdom fills the next Circle of God, the mandala. Here the six points of the entwined triangles represent the integration of Heaven and Earth. The triangle that points down to earth is woven with the triangle that points to God. By focusing on this shape you lift the veils between dimensions and begin to truly see. You are in contact with the Spiritual Hierarchy and this vision is then transformed to wisdom as it expresses through you into the world.

As you use this Sacred Tool
you are training to become a great spiritual teacher.

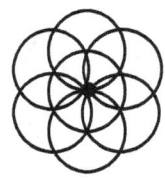

Revelation
The Key to your Crown Portal of Power
in Radiant Violet

(You may color in this symbol yourself)

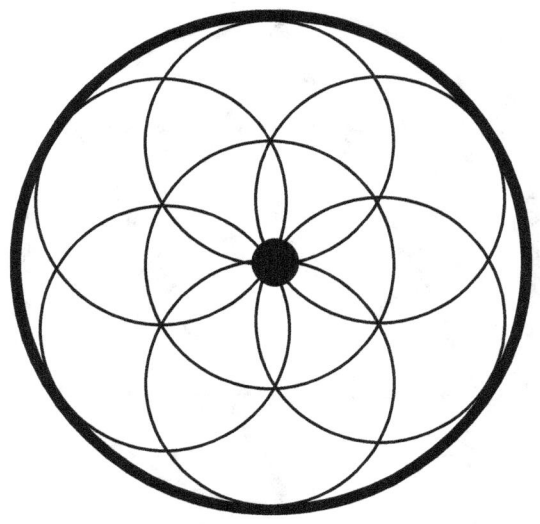

**"I am ready for God to be revealed.
All is Spirit."**

Gaze upon the blossoming lotus! The final Sacred Symbol moves and pulsates and lives. The seven circles, representing the seven levels of your Soul's evolvement rotate around the center point, you. As you focus on this shape your mind is filled with the memory of your completed lessons. The experiences of all your many lives coalesce into this one instant of Revelation. Your use of all the preceding Sacred Symbols is crowned by this final experience. Here full balance and expression is found. The keys to your Portals of Power, these Sacred Symbols, have opened the gates to Heaven. . .

*You meet God,
And God is You!*

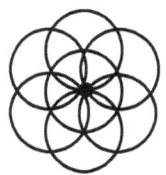

Sacred Touch

For yourself and others

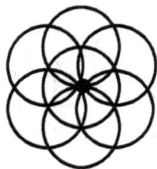

"My body is of service for a while. . .to keep its usefulness while it can serve. . ."

A Course in Miracles

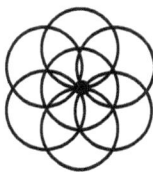

Sacred Touch throughout Time...

As the Knights of the Round Table gathered in Merlin's cave, the sorcerer raised his arms. Extending from his right hand was a short stick, his magic wand. The knights watched with both awe and unease as Merlin began to wave his wand high in the air, creating graceful and complex forms, almost visible, but powerfully felt by all. The room seemed to sizzle and spark with power...

Deep within the jungle growth a clearing had been created. Small huts circled the clearing and a group of almost naked men, women and children waited near one. An obviously ill woman lay on a mat outside the door. As she painfully waited, the shaman emerged from within. He was painted white, with beads and small bones strung around his neck, wrists and ankles. He squatted next to the woman and as he began to chant he shook a rattle in complex movements over the woman. The people watched as the illness lifted like a black mist from the woman's body...

The Chinese Emperor called the doctor forward. The young prince was ill, and so the doctor began his examination. After careful analysis he noticed an imbalance in the Toaist principle of yin and yang within the young man. He prescribed herbs, and small needles to be placed in certain parts of the boy's body to shift and balance the chi energy that runs along the fourteen major meridians in the subtle body...

Downtown, in a major hospital an older man anxiously awaits surgery. To assure the best possible success he has called upon some extra help. A middle aged women enters. She is one of the health professionals at the hospital who has also been trained as a Reiki Master and will aid in the healing process. As the the man rests on his bed the woman prays quietly and then lovingly begins to draw complex, weaving patterns over the man's body with her hands. Peace settles on the room...

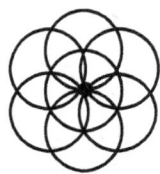

Your Metabody. . .

Everyone is aware of their physical body within which they are encased. However, few are aware of the more etheric body within which the physical body resides. This metaphysical body, which I have shortened to call the metabody, is made up of a subtler, more refined form of energy which the Hindu tradition calls *prana* and the Oriental tradition calls *chi*.

This metabody contains channels along which the Life Force flows connecting your spiritual Self with your physical body. Up and down the inner channel of your metabody, called the *shushumna*, flows Life Force, usually referred to in Sanskrit as the *Kundalini*. Hindu and Oriental medicine has acknowledged the metabody and its channels of Life Force for thousands of years. Acupuncturists trained in Oriental techniques utilize the meridians of flowing *chi* that radiate from the metabody into and along the physical body when they insert and manipulate small needles through the skin.

Also contained within the metabody, and placed along the inner channel, are seven Portals of Power, the *chakras* already mentioned. These seven major energy centers are superimposed over your physical body near important organs and glands. Through the interweaving of the metabody and the physical body these energy centers share Life Force with the corresponding areas of the physical body.

As you work to cleanse and balance your body, you must also work to cleanse and balance your metabody. Since your metabody and your mind are on the same level, it will be in the mind where the work of healing your metabody takes place.

As you balance and strengthen the flow of Life Force in your metabody this energy surge will pulsate powerfully up and down your inner channel, or *shushumna*, on which your Portals of Power are found. The cleansing process will include opening each of the Portals to allow more and more Life Force through them into your physical body, directly affecting its health and vitality.

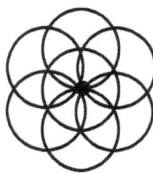

Awakening the Kundalini. . .

During a cleansing process the energy will shift within the Portals of Power and along the meridians of *chi* energy that extend from the *shushumna* throughout the rest of your body. This can be felt in surprising ways within your physical body that are not always comfortable.

When the empowering of Life Force and opening of the Portals of Power is accompanied by your spiritual acceptance of the Call from the Spiritual Masters of the Hierarchy, the shifting of energy is profound, powerful and tumultuous. This is referred to as *"awakening the Kundalini"* and is not to be attempted without experienced help, training, knowledge and a heightened sense of responsibility.

It is important and comforting to know that as you work with the Sacred Symbols they prepare you for an awakened *Kundalini* by helping to carefully open, balance, and empower your Portals of Power, strengthening Life Force within your inner channel. ***AND IT IS DONE IN A PERFECTLY SAFE AND GENTLE FASHION.***

They have been designed so that as you work with each Sacred Symbol you are anchored in a protected harbor by the Hierarchy, so that the possibly violent inner storm that sometimes accompanies the rush of *Kundalini* energy will not harm you.

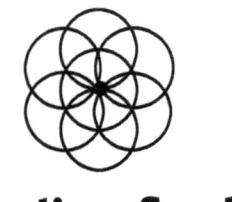

Healing Hands

Using Sacred Touch

From your subtle body flows a constant stream of energy through each Portal of Power, which then passes through bridges and then along pathways, called meridians by acupuncturists, into and along your physical body, thus increasing your well being. You can help strengthen this flow of Life Force by using the power of touch since these energy bridges also send power out through your extremities. You can, therefore, transmit energy through your hands and fingers forging a healing connection between you and another, and even with yourself.

The following will instruct you on how to move your hands over your own or another's body. Since the metabody extends a great distance beyond and around the physical body, you will be drawing within the subtle energy field of the metabody. You will be manifesting the powerful and creatively healing power of the yantras, The Sacred Symbols.

As you begin to work with Sacred Touch you will be opening, cleansing and balancing each of your Portals of Power. You will be enhancing the flow of life force along your inner subtle channels. All of this will happen within the metabody and will then flow into your physical body.

Each person will respond in his own unique fashion to the shifts of energy that occur when Portals of Power are stimulated. Some may feel more awake, others more tired. Mild aches or pains may occur along the neck, back, hips and thighs. Energy is shifting and growing in power, so this is quite normal.

Emotions and memories may emerge, sometime surprisingly. The inner process of bringing hidden issues to the surface of the mind, accompanied by the wisdom to guide you, is also growing. Be confident that the mind and the body are dealing correctly with this process.

Should any physical or emotional problem surface in a form and manner that worries you, do not hesitate to talk with a specialist about this issue that has now manifested. *Remember, the techniques offered here are to facilitate healing and are not to replace medical help that may be a necessary part of your recovery and general mental and physical health.*

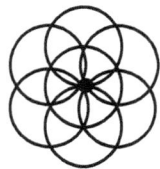

To implement healing and help alleviate fear, you must understand the relationship between your metabody and your physical body. We have begun to introduce some of the terms, concepts and functions of both these levels. But most important of all must be your understanding of the spiritual purpose behind all of what we discuss.

The spiritual purpose is, has been and always will be healing - the healing of yourself, of others, of the Universe. As long as there is one twinge of pain, fear or anger held within the heart of any expression of life, the Life Force and Divine Will is thwarted from its full experience.

Your responsibility will be to understand your own part, learn how to do it perfectly and then BE it. Healing is never accomplished in a vacuum, and so you help others in order to be helped - heal others in order to be healed.

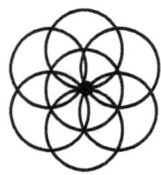

Instructions for Using Sacred Touch

. . .for yourself or others

You may use Sacred Touch on yourself or others by simply holding your hands, palms down, over each Portal of Power and tracing a Sacred Symbol over each Portal of Power, either in the air above the body, or directly on the body itself.

Remember to always draw the circle first in a clockwise direction and then add the appropriate Sacred Symbol for that Portal of Power within the circle you have just drawn.

In this way you will be invoking the Sacred Yantra of Om and drawing forth the power of each Sacred Symbol through the chakra, bringing healing from the subtle levels into the physical.

You may wish to begin by "grounding" the other person by gently holding each of their feet in one of your hands for 30 seconds and then placing your hands on either side of the person's head and holding gently for another 30 seconds.

Continue by "washing" the aura. You can do this by placing both your hands palms down over the person by his feet and with a flowing motion, move your hands over the body from feet to head. Do this three times, washing the aura from feet to head.

You are now ready to apply Sacred Touch.

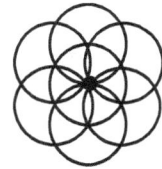

Root Portal of Power

Begin by tracing a circle over the Root Portal chanting the mantra OM as you do so. Then hold your hands steady at the center of the circle and repeat the prayer of protection for this Symbol changing it to the third person as follows, "You open to your Divine Self, and feel the love of God in you and around you."

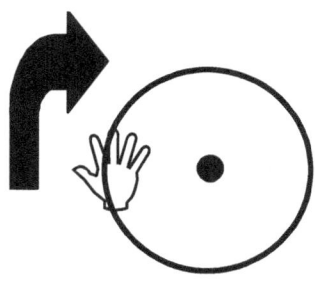

Navel Portal of Power

Once more trace a circle, but this time over the Navel Portal and chant the mantra OM as you do so. As you then trace a vertical line from top to bottom and then a horizontal line from left to right, repeat the prayer for protection as follows, "You open to balance in your life. You feel the flow of power though you."

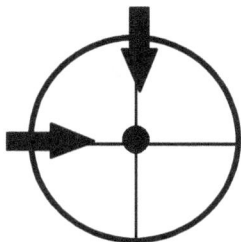

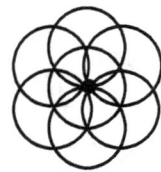

Solar Plexus Portal of Power

Now trace a circle over the Solar Plexus chanting OM. Trace a triangle within by starting with the left point, moving up to the point, down to the right point and then across to the left. Repeat the prayer of protection as follows, "You integrate and grow through your experiences. You are beginning to truly understand."

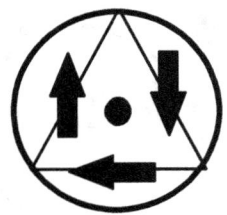

Heart Portal of Power

Trace a circle once more, this time over the Heart Portal as you chant OM. Trace the square within the circle by starting at the top left corner moving across to the right corner, down to the right corner and across to the left, and up to the left top. Repeat the prayer for protection as follows, "Your mind opens to wholeness and health. You are being reborn each moment."

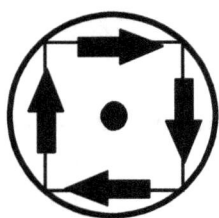

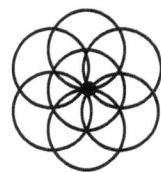

Throat Portal of Power

Trace a circle and chant OM over the Throat Portal. Begin the five pointed star at the top point and move down to the center, across to the right point, back to the center, then down to the lower right point, back to the center, now down to the left lower point and back to the center, then across to the left point and back to the center and then up to the top point. Repeat the prayer for protection as follows, " You communicate and share love with all. You are God's servant."

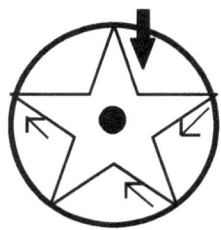

Forehead Portal of Power

Trace the circle and chant OM over the Forehead Portal. First trace the triangle that points to heaven by starting at the left point, moving up to the top then across to the right and back to the left. From this same point start the triangle pointing to earth by moving across from the left point to the right point, down to the lowest point and then up again to the left point. Repeat the prayer of protection as follows, " Wisdom is yours and you know. Serenity fills your days and nights."

Trace on top of each other

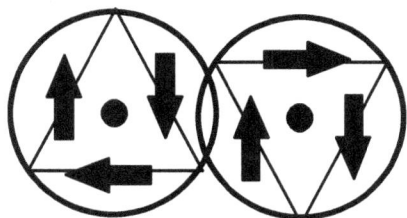

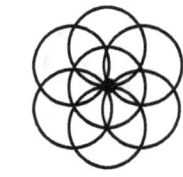

Crown Portal of Power

Now trace the last circle over the Crown Portal as you chant OM. Begin tracing the seven inner circles by tracing the first one at the top right, tracing a second circle at the right, then another circle near the bottom right, another at bottom left, another at the left and then another at the top left, then a final small circle in the center. Repeat the prayer for protection as follows, "You are ready for God to be revealed. All is Spirit. All is Spirit. All is Spirit."

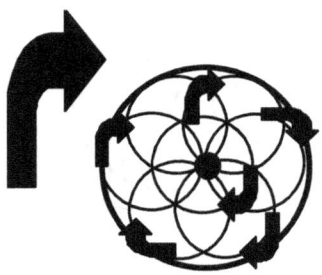

To complete this healing treatment you may once more hold the person's head for 30 seconds and then the feet for 30 seconds. Announce quietly that you are done, and wait a few moments for the person to "awaken".

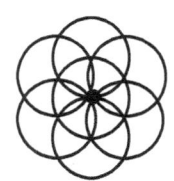

The Workbook

7 Months of Daily Lessons

. . .for your Body

. . .for your Relationships

. . .for your Mind

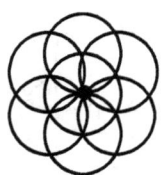

"An untrained mind can accomplish nothing."

A Course in Miracles

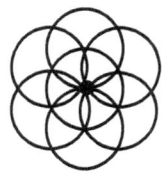

Karma — Life's Original Health Club

From your first breath in the delivery room your Personal Trainer is on your case coaching you through the cross training of life. Sometimes like a drill sergeant and sometimes like a nurturing mother, Karma leads you through sit-ups, iron pumping, and laps, building stamina and strength for your Soul's journey.

You may think you have some control over your life experiences, but think again! Your personal training program was already designed way before you were born. I know it seems unlikely but, yes, you had a willing part in its design. However, on a day to day basis in this lifetime, mister, you gotta do what you're told!

Your life is perfectly planned to include just the right combinations of challenges and rewards to balance your inner growth process. You, your parents and siblings agreed to be together because of the personality conflicts you offered each other, not in spite of them. You are all a part of a karmic group following each other, through lifetime after lifetime, constantly reversing roles.

Each of us carries around a karmic VISA card that is usually maxed out. And so each lifetime gives us another opportunity to pay down our debt. In fact, we have charged so much against humanity in the past that it is usually impossible to pay down our karmic loan totally in one lifetime, and so our karmic training program includes only just the right combinations of relationships and experiences to focus on just a few parts of our debt.

For some this may seem depressing. But for others this perspective offers a reason for the seeming tragedies in the world, and purpose to each person's life - to help bring forgiveness, peace and healing into each moment of each day. This is the only payment necessary, and what a great way to give and receive at the same time.

The following Workbook is designed to guide you through your personal training program smoothly and easily. The Workbook offers a spiraling process for healing the issues around your body, your relationships and your thought patterns. You will spend seven weeks healing these three areas from the perspective of the Root Portal of Power and then progress to the next seven weeks focused on the Navel Portal of Power, the Solar Plexus Portal, and so on until the issues attached to all seven Portals have been addressed. Thus the opportunity for dysfunctional habits to be changed to healthy ones will be offered again and again. Simply remember to follow the directions and. . .

. . .face each day with the enthusiasm of the health nut - and reap the rewards of spiritual progress. For as you sprint through life the runner's high can be yours eternally!

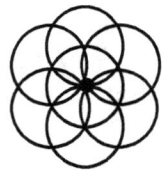

"You have need for the symbols of the world a while."

A Course in Miracles

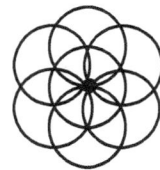

Your Root Portal of Power
Week One
Opening to Divinity and Your body

Prayer of Protection, repeat daily for the next four weeks:
"I open to my Divine Self and feel the love of God in me and around me."

Remember to meditate on all Seven Sacred Symbols each and every day.
These are the powerful tools given to you to accelerate your Soul's progress.

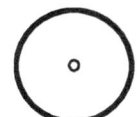 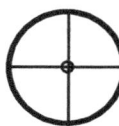 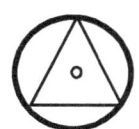 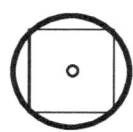  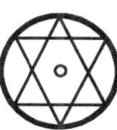 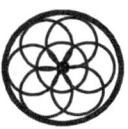

DAY ONE: Stand in front a full length mirror and observe your front and back and affirm, "This is a sacred tool I must honor."

DAY TWO: Look at and observe carefully one or both of your hands for 3-5 minutes. What miraculous insights do you gain? Write them down if you wish.

DAY THREE: Observe the physical world around you, the Earth's body - her sky, her natural vegetation, her air that you breath. Give thanks to this lovely mother.

DAY FOUR: Ask yourself, "Where is God?" then list all the physical aspects of God's reflections that you can see.

DAY FIVE: Referring to the previous days' list say silently or out loud to each physical manifestation of Divinity you meet (yourself, your meals, your home, Mother Earth), "Your Divinity blesses me."

DAY SIX: Referring once more to your list, say to each physical manifestation of Divinity you meet, "My Divinity blesses you."

DAY SEVEN: Review all that you have experienced and learned this week. Set aside an extra 14 minutes during the day to meditate on the Seven Sacred Symbols and open your heart with gratitude to their healing power.

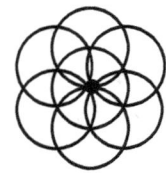

Your Root Portal of Power
Week Two
Opening to Divinity and Your Relationships

Remember to meditate on all Seven Sacred Symbols each and every day.
These are the powerful tools given to you to accelerate your Soul's progress.

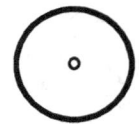 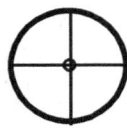 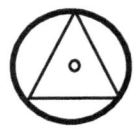 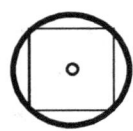  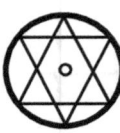 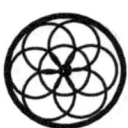

DAY ONE: Make a list of the people in your life who you enjoy thinking about. Look each name and say, "I've seen your Divinity."

DAY TWO: Make a list of the people in your life that seem to bring pain when thought about. Look at each name and say, "I need Divine Help to see your Divinity."

DAY THREE: As you interact with each person in your life today, say to them silently, "I honor the Divinity in you."

DAY FOUR: As you interact with each person in your life today, say to them silently, "Your Divinity honors me."

DAY FIVE: Look once more at the list of people in your life that seem to cause pain when thought of and say to each name, "If I deny your Divinity, I am denying my own."

DAY SIX: Allow your mind to think of all the people you love and all those you still have difficulty with and say to each as you think of them, "Divine Love fills us, connects us and brings us peace."

DAY SEVEN: Review all that you have experienced and learned this week. Set aside an extra 14 minutes during the day to meditate on the Seven Sacred Symbols and open your heart with gratitude to their healing power.

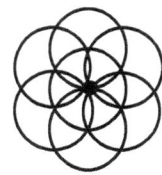

Your Root Portal of Power
Week Three
Opening to Divinity and Your Mind

Prayer of Protection
"I open to my Divine Self and feel the love of God in me and around me."

Remember to meditate on all Seven Sacred Symbols each and every day.
These are the powerful tools given to you to accelerate your Soul's progress.

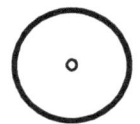 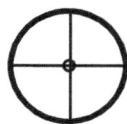 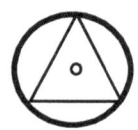 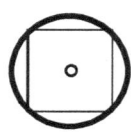  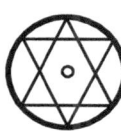 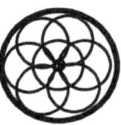

DAY ONE: Observe the flow of your thoughts today and ask yourself as often as possible, "Are these thoughts reflecting my Divinity?"

DAY TWO: Begin your day by stating, "I wish my thoughts to reflect my Divinity," then observe and monitor how closely your thoughts follow your statement.

DAY THREE: Begin your day by stating, "My mind is a Divine tool and I place it in Divine Hands." Monitor your thoughts today, and when necessary repeat today's statement to correct obviously UNdivine thoughts.

DAY FOUR: Set aside 15-30 minutes today. Write down any and all pleasant, inspired and Divine thoughts, stories, poems or perhaps just words that occur to you. Enjoy what your mind has created.

DAY FIVE: Begin your day by stating, "My Divine Mind is filled with Divine Thoughts." Let your mind guide you to see, feel and experience Divinity all day.

DAY SIX: Notice the Divine Thought that fills you and your world and affirm as often as possible today, "Divine Thought is all that truly is."

DAY SEVEN: Review all that you have experienced and learned this week. Set aside an extra 14 minutes during the day to meditate on the Seven Sacred Symbols and open your heart with gratitude to their healing power.

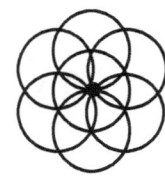

Your Root Portal of Power
Week Four
Opening to Divinity and Love

This week will be a time of rest, a time for digestion and assimilation. All you need do each day is spend an extra 14 minutes meditating on the seven Sacred Symbols.

As you spend this extra time each day in meditation allow the Sacred Symbols themselves to work for you. You need not do anything but look at them. The rest will be done for you, for you will be using these times as prayerful invitations for remembrance of the Divinity and Love that is yours

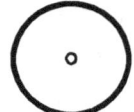 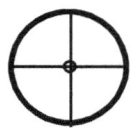 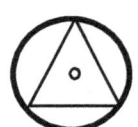 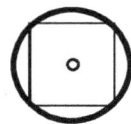  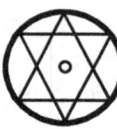 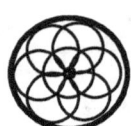

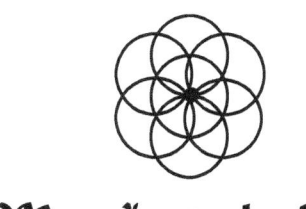

My Journal Notes

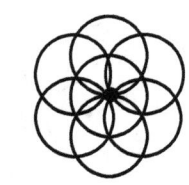

My Journal Notes

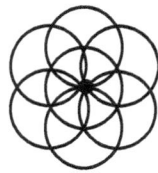

Your Navel Portal of Power
Week One
Opening to Balance and Your Body

Prayer of Protection for the next four weeks:
"All is in balance in my life. I feel the flow of Power through me."

Remember to meditate on all Seven Sacred Symbols each and every day.
These are the powerful tools given to you to accelerate your Soul's progress.

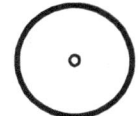 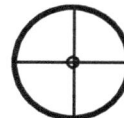 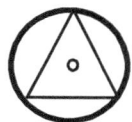 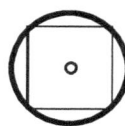  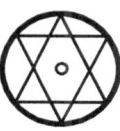 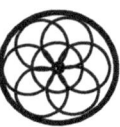

DAY ONE: Today simply observe your sleeping, eating, working, playing and resting rhythm. At the end of the day write down a simple outline of this rhythm.

DAY TWO: Look at last night's outline and decide which areas need to be increased or decreased to gain a more balanced daily rhythm. Begin to DO what you decide.

DAY THREE: First thing in the morning affirm, "I desire harmony and balance to be reflected in my eating habits. I, therefore, will bless and respect all the foods I eat."

DAY FOUR: First thing in the morning affirm, "I desire harmony and balance in the rhythm between worktime and playtime. Both are times for expressing the Will of God and I will honor this."

DAY FIVE: First thing in the morning affirm, "I desire the harmony and balance that comes from honoring my sleep needs. This is the time when God replenishes me through my subconscious."

DAY SIX: Today I review once more the full schedule of my daily rhythms and decide on the changes that are needed. "I bring balance to my body by desiring God's Harmony to flow through the rhythms of my day."

DAY SEVEN: Review all that you have experienced and learned this week. Set aside an extra 14 minutes during the day to meditate on the Seven Sacred Symbols and open your heart with gratitude to their healing power.

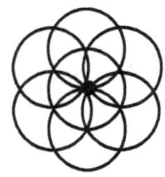

Your Navel Portal of Power
Week Two
Opening to Balance and Your Relationships

Prayer of Protection
"All is in balance in my life. I feel the flow of Power through me."

*Remember to meditate on all Seven Sacred Symbols each and every day.
These are the powerful tools given to you to accelerate your Soul's progress.*

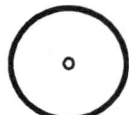 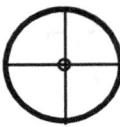 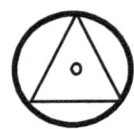 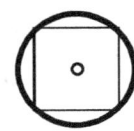  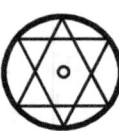 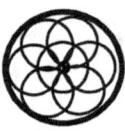

DAY ONE: Choose a time today when you can sit quietly and list the names of the relationships in your life. Group them under the following headings: family, friends, co-workers, lovers, enemies. You can place a name in several categories if its fits.

DAY TWO: Review your list of relationships and notice any glaring imbalances, (no names in one area, one or two names that overlap several headings.) Then affirm, "I will acknowledge ALL the people I deal with today as important, and honor this."

DAY THREE: First thing in the morning affirm, "I will see all the relationships in my life in one category - beloved friends." Say this silently to everyone you see or think of.

DAY FOUR: All through the day, should you notice obsessive focusing on one relationship either a loved one or an enemy, affirm, "You are just one gift in my life and I must honor all the others."

DAY FIVE: All through the day as you think of or deal with your relationships affirm, "I am a gift to each of you and give myself equally."

DAY SIX: Review your original outline that categorized the relationships in your life, add any new names and write next to each one - You are equally important to me.

DAY SEVEN: Review all that you have experienced and learned this week. Set aside an extra 14 minutes during the day to meditate on the Seven Sacred Symbols and open your heart with gratitude to their healing power.

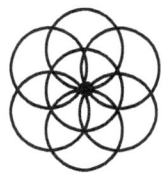

Your Navel Portal of Power
Week Three
Opening to Balance and Your Mind

Prayer of Protection
"All is in balance in my life. I feel the flow of Power through me."

*Remember to meditate on all Seven Sacred Symbols each and every day.
These are the powerful tools given to you to accelerate your Soul's progress.*

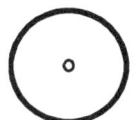 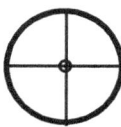 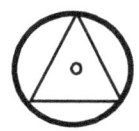 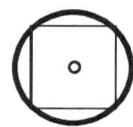  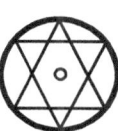 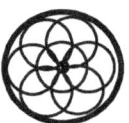

DAY ONE: Today observe the flow of your thoughts and emotions. Notice the percetnage of time you are happy, excited, worried, angry, depressed.

DAY TWO: First thing today affirm, "I will feel emotions today. When they are pleasant I will say, 'thank you', and when they are unpleasant I will say, 'I can feel differently about this.'

DAY THREE: Real mental balance comes from desiring God's Mind to guide all thoughts, so affirm today, "I will let God guide all my thinking today."

DAY FOUR: Remind youself all through the day, "I must be honest with how I feel." Make a point of labeling your feelings today as painful or pleasant.

DAY FIVE: Affirm all through the day, "I will feel emotions and not feel gulty when they are unpleasant, but I DO NOT HAVE TO HOLD ON TO THEM."

DAY SIX: Remind yourself that you are the author of your feelings and affirm, "My mind is balanced when I choose to let God guide my mind. I can learn to change unpleasant feelings to pleasant ones."

DAY SEVEN: Review all that you have experienced and learned this week. Set aside an extra 14 minutes during the day to meditate on the Seven Sacred Symbols and open your heart with gratitude to their healing power.

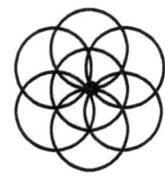

Your Navel Portal of Power
Week Four
Opening to Balance and Power

Prayer of Protection
"All is in balance in my life. I feel the flow of Power through me."

This week will be a time of rest, a time for digestion and assimilation. All you need do each day is spend an extra 14 minutes meditating on the seven Sacred Symbols.

As you spend this extra time each day in meditation allow the Sacred Symbols themselves to work for you. You need not do anything but look at them. The rest will be done for you, for you will be using these times as prayerful invitations for remembrance of the Balance and Power that is yours.

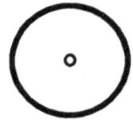 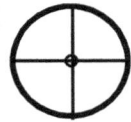 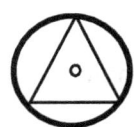 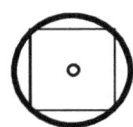  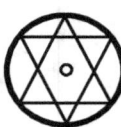 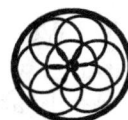

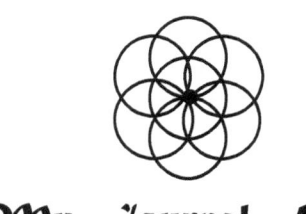

My Journal Notes

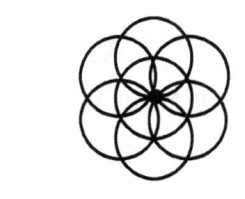

My Journal Notes

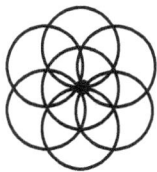

Your Solar Plexus Portal of Power
Week One
Opening to Integration and Your Body

Prayer of Protection for the next four weeks:
"I integrate and grow through my experiences. I am beginning to truly understand."

Remember to meditate on all Seven Sacred Symbols each and every day.
These are the powerful tools given to you to accelerate your Soul's progress.

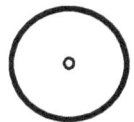 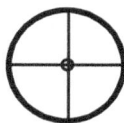 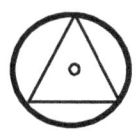 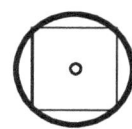  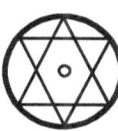 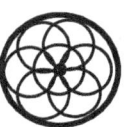

DAY ONE: Your body can only work smoothly when all aspects of physical health are respected. Throughout the day affirm, "I will respect all aspects of my physical needs."

DAY TWO: Take the time throughout the day to observe how your eating habits are directly affecting your levels of energy. At the end of the day review your observations and decide to make changes where necessary.

DAY THREE: As you awake this morning reflect back on your sleep cycle and observe it correlating to your eating habits Would eating more or less or different foods before you go to bed enhance your sleep? Plan the necessary changes for the nights ahead.

DAY FOUR: Take the time today to review the balance between your physical activities and your times of relaxation. Replan this taking into account your eating habits and sleep needs.

DAY FIVE: Spend some time today reviewing your basic health issues. If you are due for a medical or dental check-up, make the appointments. Delay no more!

DAY SIX: Affirm throughout the day, "My body is a perfectly working machine. I will use it for God's work."

DAY SEVEN: Review all that you have experienced and learned this week. Set aside an extra 14 minutes during the day to meditate on the Seven Sacred Symbols and

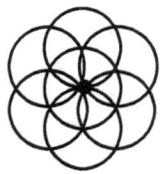

Your Solar Plexus Portal of Power
Week Two
Opening to Integration and Your Relationships

Prayer of Protection
"I integrate and grow through my experiences. I am beginning to truly understand."

Remember to meditate on all Seven Sacred Symbols each and every day.
These are the powerful tools given to you to accelerate your Soul's progress.

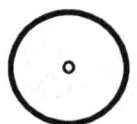 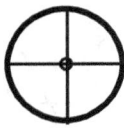 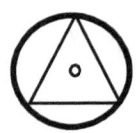 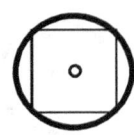  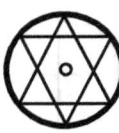 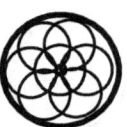

DAY ONE: Begin this week by affirming throughout the day, "All my relationships are an integral part of my growth and life."

DAY TWO: As the day unfolds notice how each person you interact with helps you understand more about yourself and others. Keep a journal of these encounters and what they teach you.

DAY THREE: As the day unfolds observe how you are a part of all other people's learning experiences. Add these encounters and the lessons taught by you to others into the journal begun yesterday.

DAY FOUR: Set aside a quiet time to review your past relationships. Notice how you affected them and they you and add these observations to your journal.

DAY FIVE: Sometime during the day sit quietly reaching for the "silence" affirming, "I am an integrated part of my relationship to God."

DAY SIX: Affirm throughout the day, "I am an integral part of all my relationships, as they are with me."

DAY SEVEN: Review all that you have experienced and learned this week. Set aside an extra 14 minutes during the day to meditate on the Seven Sacred Symbols and open your heart with gratitude to their healing power.

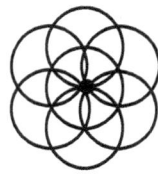

Your Solar Plexus Portal of Power
Week Three
Opening to Integration and Your Mind

Prayer of Protection
"I integrate and grow through my experiences. I am beginning to truly understand."

Remember to meditate on all Seven Sacred Symbols each and every day.
These are the powerful tools given to you to accelerate your Soul's progress.

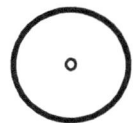 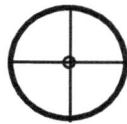 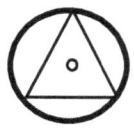 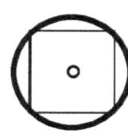  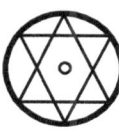 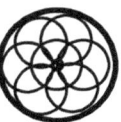

DAY ONE: Use the day for observing the flow of your thoughts. Notice what triggers each train of thought.

DAY TWO: Make distinctions today between mood and thought. What comes first, the mood or the thought; and which seems to stimulate the continuation of the other?

DAY THREE:Affirm throughout the day, "Whenever my mood is not happy or peaceful, "I align my thoughts with God's Thought insead."

DAY FOUR: Begin to integrate all your thoughts and moods by affirming throughout the day, "God will guide my thinking and my mood will follow."

DAY FIVE: Use today to continue disciplining your mind so that real integration of God's Thought and your thoughts can occur by not allowing any unhappy mood or train of thought to continue unchecked.

DAY SIX: Your mind and its thoughts are always integrated and never random. They are either aligned with God or not. Choose for alignment by affirming, "God's Thought is all I want."

DAY SEVEN: Review all that you have experienced and learned this week. Set aside an extra 14 minutes during the day to meditate on the Seven Sacred Symbols and open your heart with gratitude to their healing power.

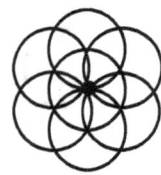

Your Solar Plexus Portal of Power
Week Four
Opening to Integration and Understanding

Prayer of Protection
"I integrate and grow through my experiences. I am beginning to truly understand."

This week will be a time of rest, a time for digestion and assimilation. All you need do each day is spend an extra 14 minutes meditating on the seven Sacred Symbols.

As you spend this extra time each day in meditation allow the Sacred Symbols themselves to work for you. You need not do anything but look at them. The rest will be done for you, for you will be using these times as prayerful invitations for remembrance of the Intergration and Understanding that is yours.

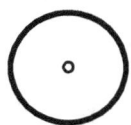 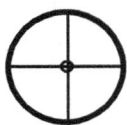 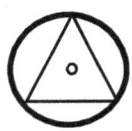 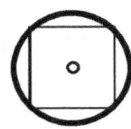  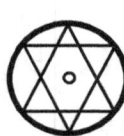 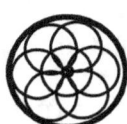

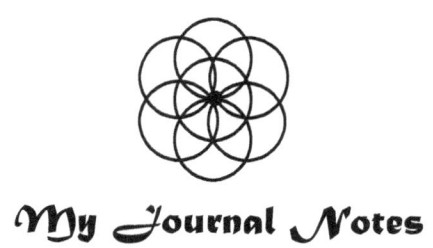

My Journal Notes

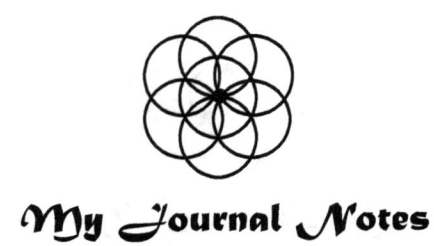

My Journal Notes

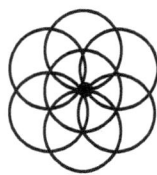

Your Heart Portal of Power

Week One
Opening to Health and Your Body

Prayer of Protection for the next four weeks:
"My mind opens to wholeness and health. I am being reborn each moment."

Remember to meditate on all Seven Sacred Symbols each and every day.
These are the powerful tools given to you to accelerate your Soul's progress.

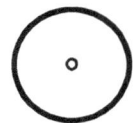 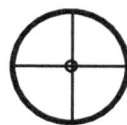 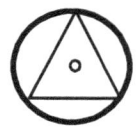 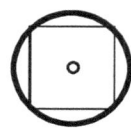  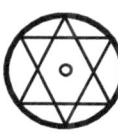 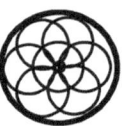

DAY ONE: Take some time today to list the parts of your body that you do not like. Next to each part write, "I forgive you for not being the way I think you should be."

DAY TWO: Review yesterdays' list and then as your day unfolds observe the workings of these parts of your body and affirm, "I accept you just the way you are."

DAY THREE: Sometime during the day stand in front of a mirror and as you look at each part of your body affirm, "You are a perfect tool for God's work and I am grateful."

DAY FOUR: Take some time today in a natural environment to contemplate Mother Earth and your gratitude to Her. Affirm, "I am a part of you and you a part of me."

DAY FIVE: Throughout the day affirm, "My body is whole for it is connected to Everything."

DAY SIX: Take some time today to sit quietly and feel the flowing integration of all your body functions and your connection to the Earth. Affirm, "We are whole."

DAY SEVEN: Review all that you have experienced and learned this week. Set aside an extra 14 minutes during the day to meditate on the Seven Sacred Symbols and open your heart with gratitude to their healing power.

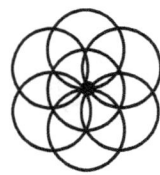

Your Heart Portal of Power
Week Two
Opening to Health and Your Relationships

Remember to meditate on all Seven Sacred Symbols each and every day.
These are the powerful tools given to you to accelerate your Soul's progress.

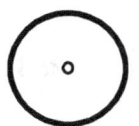 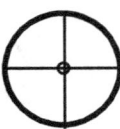 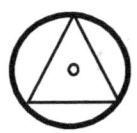 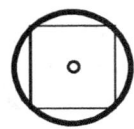  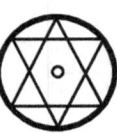 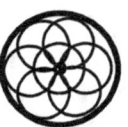

DAY ONE: Begin this week by offering this prayer, "I wish to feel healing in all my relationships."

DAY TWO: Make a list of all your on-going relationships. Next to each name write, "I want to experience healing with you."

DAY THREE: Take some time first thing in the morning to think about your relationships. As each one comes to mind affirm, "God will show me how to forgive you of any weaknesses or faults. I do this for my own healing."

DAY FOUR: Take some time first thing in the morning to once more think about each relationship, this time affirming with each one, "God will show me how to forgive myself of any weakness or fault. I do this for the healing of our relationship."

DAY FIVE: As your day unfolds affirm silently with each relationship, "I want to see our wholeness by opening my mind to forgiveness of you and me."

DAY SIX: Affirm throughout the day, "I may not know how to forgive myself and others, but God will show me why I can be healed."

DAY SEVEN: Review all that you have experienced and learned this week. Set aside an extra 14 minutes during the day to meditate on the Seven Sacred Symbols and open your heart with gratitude to their healing power.

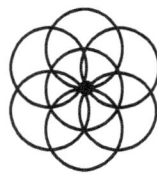

Your Heart Portal of Power
Week Three
Opening to Health and Your Mind

Remember to meditate on all Seven Sacred Symbols each and every day.
These are the powerful tools given to you to accelerate your Soul's progress.

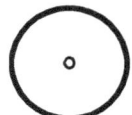 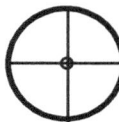 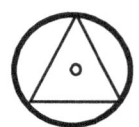 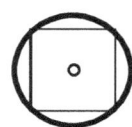  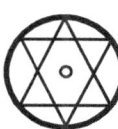 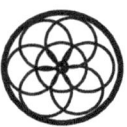

DAY ONE: Take some time this morning to sit quietly following the flow of your thoughts. As you become aware of each thought affirm, "This thought leads to wholeness or is in need of forgiveness."

DAY TWO: Once more allow some quiet time in the morning for you to observe your mind. As each thought passes, affirm, "I turn this thought over to God so that my mind will be filled with healing."

DAY THREE: As your day unfolds, observe your thoughts and correct any unforgiving thoughts by saying, "I want my mind to be healed and so I request forgiving insight."

DAY FOUR: Spend at least an extra 14 minutes today in quiet contemplation of the oneness of your mind with God's Mind, affirming, "When I share God's Thoughts I am healed."

DAY FIVE: Affirm throughout the day, "I wish only to have thoughts of healing, wholeness and forgiveness."

DAY SIX: Affirm throughout the day, "My mind is filled with forgiving thoughts and so I offer healing to myself and the world."

DAY SEVEN: Review all that you have experienced and learned this week. Set aside an extra 14 minutes during the day to meditate on the Seven Sacred Symbols and open your heart with gratitude to their healing power.

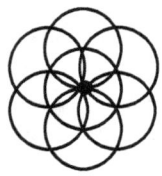

𝒀our 𝕳eart 𝕻ortal of 𝕻ower
Week Four
Opening to Health and Rebirth

𝕻rayer of 𝕻rotection
"My mind opens to wholeness and health. I am being reborn each moment."

     This week will be a time of rest, a time for digestion and assimilation. All you need do each day is spend an extra 14 minutes meditating on the seven Sacred Symbols.

     As you spend this extra time each day in meditation allow the Sacred Symbols themselves to work for you. You need not do anything but look at them. The rest will be done for you, for you will be using these times as prayerful invitations for remembrance of the Health and Rebirth that is yours.

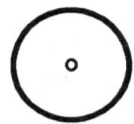 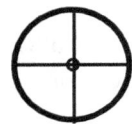 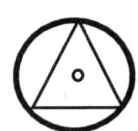 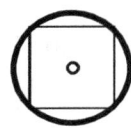  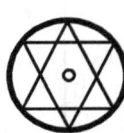 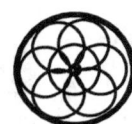

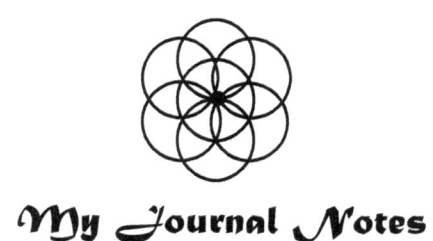

My Journal Notes

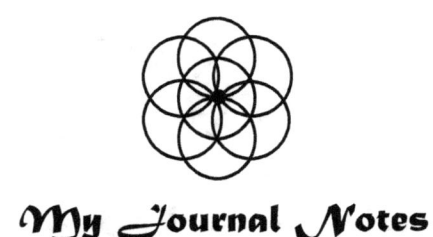

My Journal Notes

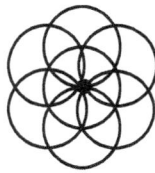

Your Throat Portal of Power
Week One
Opening to Communication and Your Body
Prayer of Protection for the next four weeks:
"I communicate and share love with all. I am God's servant."

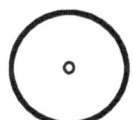 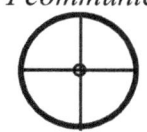 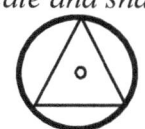 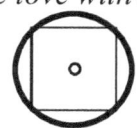  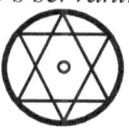 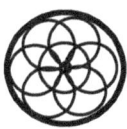

DAY ONE: Your body is a tool, and therefore, must be given the correct instructions. Affirm throughout the day, "I am responsible for my body."

DAY TWO: Your body is a responsive machine. Thus, you must listen to its feedback in order to direct it properly. Take time throughout the day to observe the messages your body is giving you.

DAY THREE: Take some time first thing in the morning, and then again twice more throughout the day to sit quietly and listen to your body. Is it comfortable, hungry, cold, feeling discomfort anywhere? Make note of this feedback, writing comments down if necessary.

DAY FOUR: Begin to examine how you support your body. Do you eat appropriately? Do you exercise regularly? Do you get enough sleep? If you have physical discomfort that requires medical attention, do you seek professional advice? Learn to listen to your body's needs.

DAY FIVE: Spend at least 15 minutes today quietly resting and attuning your body to a peaceful mind.

DAY SIX: Spend at least 15 minutes today attuning your body to the rhythms and messages from the Earth. Affirm thought the day, "I listen to my body's rhythms and align them to the Earth's."

DAY SEVEN: Review all that you have experienced and learned this week. Set aside an extra 14 minutes during the day to meditate on the Seven Sacred Symbols and open your heart with gratitude to their healing power.

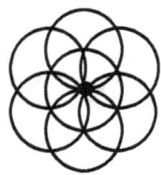

Your Throat Portal of Power
Week Two
Opening to Communication and Your Relationships
Prayer of Protection
"I communicate and share love with all. I am God's servant."

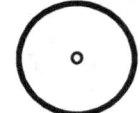 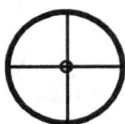 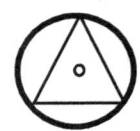 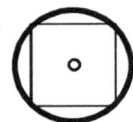  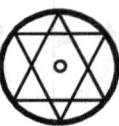 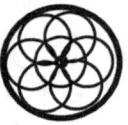

DAY ONE: Sit quietly first thing in the morning and request the ability to listen and share correctly with all your relationships. Affirm, "I want to learn effective communication."

DAY TWO: Keep a notebook handy all through the day. As you interact with each relationship take notes on what you hear using these two headings: 1 - what is said, 2 - what is meant. This a good practice for listening fully and truly and will help you respond to what is truly being asked.

DAY THREE: Once more keep a notebook with you and take notes again on what is said and what is meant. This time add your own verbal responses, as well as what you truly mean. Be honest. You are the only one seeing your notes. Discrepancy between what you say and mean needs correction.

DAY FOUR: Affirm throughout the day, I will listen fully and Irespond honestly and helpfully."

DAY FIVE: Observe your listening habits today. Notice when you don't fully listen to others by doing other activities when they are talking. Do you have a tendency to add your own ideas before you have fully heard another's? Avoid downgrading the important of another's comments. When you notice counter productive habits stop yourself immediately and listen!

DAY SIX: Sit quietly at least once today for a total of 10-15 minutes thanking all your relationships for what they communicate to you.

DAY SEVEN: Review all that you have experienced and learned this week. Set aside an extra 14 minutes during the day to meditate on the Seven Sacred Symbols and open your heart with gratitude to their healing power.

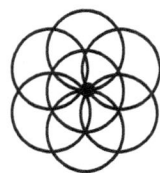

Your Throat Portal of Power
Week Three
Opening to Communication and Your Mind
Prayer of Protection

"I communicate and share love with all. I am God's servant."

Remember to meditate on all Seven Sacred Symbols each and every day.
These are the powerful tools given to you to accelerate your Soul's progress.

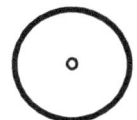 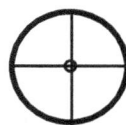 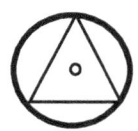 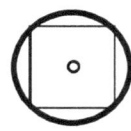  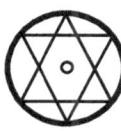 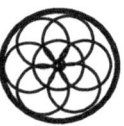

DAY ONE: Your mind is both transmitter and receiver. Affirm this by saying throughout the day, "My mind is powerful tool for communication. I will respect it."

DAY TWO: Your mind communicates its thoughts directly from your mind to all other minds instantaneously. Observe throughout the day the messages in your mind that you are sending forth.

DAY THREE: Affirm throughout the day, "I will send forth messages of support and help. I am responsible for what I communicate."

DAY FOUR: Take time in the morning to sit quietly for 10-15 minutes. Observe how busy your mind is. Begin to release this mental activity by addressing each thought with the following: "I am finished with this thought for now." You may need most of those minutes to quiet the mental activity. Silence is the first step in being able to truly hear.

DAY FIVE: Take three to four quiet times today when you can "listen to the silence". Affirm, "I wish to hear what God has to say." Note that a sense of peace may be His only response.

DAY SIX: Use the day to observe the gentle, powerful or perhaps exciting messages that you hear and that you can share solely within your mind.

DAY SEVEN: Review all that you have experienced and learned this week. Set aside an extra 14 minutes during the day to meditate on the Seven Sacred Symbols and open your heart with gratitude to their healing power.

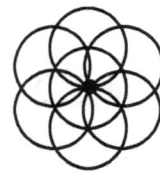

Your Throat Portal of Power
Week Four
Opening to Communication and Service

Prayer of Protection
"I communicate and share love with all. I am God's servant."

      This week will be a time of rest, a time for digestion and assimilation. All you need do each day is spend an extra 14 minutes meditating on the seven Sacred Symbols.

      As you spend this extra time each day in meditation allow the Sacred Symbols themselves to work for you. You need not do anything but look at them. The rest will be done for you, for you will be using these times as prayerful invitations for remembrance of the Commucation and Service that is yours.

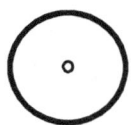 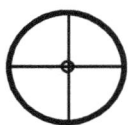 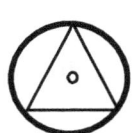 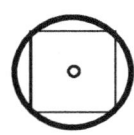  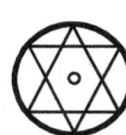 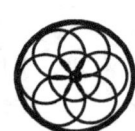

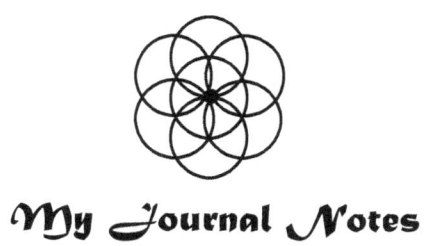

My Journal Notes

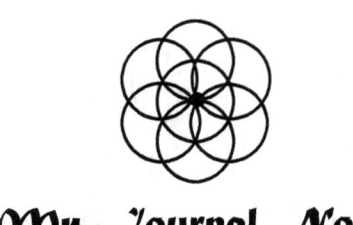

My Journal Notes

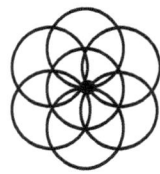

Your Forehead Portal of Power
Week One
Opening to Wisdom and Your Body

Prayer of Protection for the next four weeks:
"Wisdom is mine and I know. Serenity fills my days and nights."

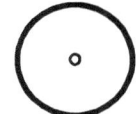 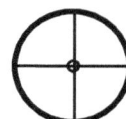 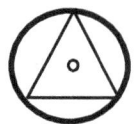 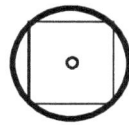  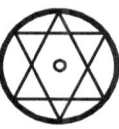 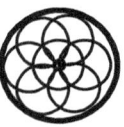

DAY ONE: Set aside 10-15 minutes some time during the day to quietly begin sensing your subtle, or metabody. You will sense it not only within you but extending about three feet around you. If you do not sense it then imagine it and this will do.

DAY TWO: Sit quietly first thing in the morning and place your hands at each of your Portals of Power, fingers of each hand facing and touching each other with palms over each area in turn. Try to sense, or imagine, the power flow that enters and extends from these areas.

DAY THREE: Once more sit quietly and visualize within you a channel of energy beginning at the base of your spine and ending at the top of your head. See this channel filled with a weaving flowing light.

DAY FOUR: Set aside quiet time once more today. Visualize the inner channel of flowing light, this time seeing each Portal of Power as a pulsating wheel of colored energy as follows: Root-red, Navel-orange, Solar Plexus-yellow, Heart-green, Throat-bright blue, Forehead-deep blue, Crown-violet.

DAY FIVE: Throughout the day affirm, "My Portals of Power are pulsating through my physical and subtle body."

DAY SIX: Throughout the day affirm, "The Sacred Cobra sends her Wisdom through each of my Portals of Power.

DAY SEVEN: Review all that you have experienced and learned this week. Set aside an extra 14 minutes during the day to meditate on the Seven Sacred Symbols and open your heart with gratitude to their healing power.

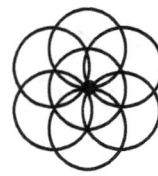

Your Forehead Portal of Power
Week Two
Opening to Wisdom and Your Relationships

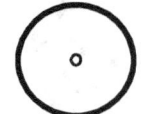 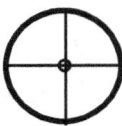 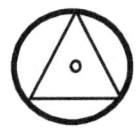 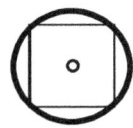  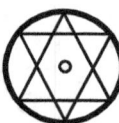 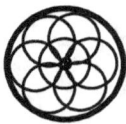

DAY ONE: As your day unfolds be aware that yours and everyone else's personal energy fields are at least three feet or more wide. This represents the body's auric field. Notice how often you are melding energy fields with others.

DAY TWO: As your day unfolds affirm silently as you meet each relationships, "We are melding our energies and gain wisdom from the contact."

DAY THREE: Take some time today to relax in a natural environment. Touch the plants, breath the air, feel the firmness of the ground and affirm, "Our energy fields are melding and we gain wisdom with the contact."

DAY FOUR: Sit quietly for 10-15 minutes some time during the day affirming, "The energy field of the world melds with my energy field." Visualize youself and the earth joined with white light.

DAY FIVE: As your day unfolds hold an inner picture of the flow of your energy field in contact with that of the people you meet and the world as a whole. Affirm, "We are one and I am filled with wisdom and knowing."

DAY SIX: Spend quiet time today affirming, "All my relationships, past, present and future are melding with me now. I am filled with their wisdom."

DAY SEVEN: Review all that you have experienced and learned this week. Set aside an extra 14 minutes during the day to meditate on the Seven Sacred Symbols and open your heart with gratitude to their healing power.

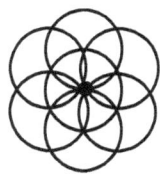

Your Forehead Portal of Power
Week Three
Opening to Wisdom and Your Mind

Prayer of Protection
"Wisdom is mine and I know. Serenity fills my days and nights."

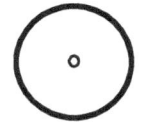 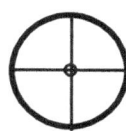 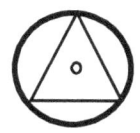 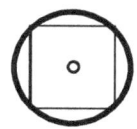  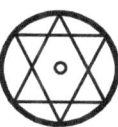 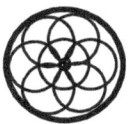

DAY ONE: Sit quietly for 10-15 minutes affirming, "My mind is one with God's Mind."

DAY TWO: Throughout the day observe your thought labeling as such, 1- these thoughts tap the Wisdom of the Universe, 2 - these thoughts block the Wisdom of the Universe.

DAY THREE: Affirm throughout the day, "I open my mind to the Wisdom of the Universe and all my thoughts will follow."

DAY FOUR: Loving thoughts connect. Unloving thoughts block. Affirm through the day, "Loving thoughts connect me with Wisdom. I choose loving thoughts."

DAY FIVE: As you make decisions and choices throughout the day, affirm, "My mind can connect with God's Mind and His Wisdom. I want this insight now."

DAY SIX: Spend 10-15 minutes quieting the mind. As you do so you are expanding your mind to enter and fill the recesses of Eternity where all Wisdom is gained. During these times your energy field expands beyond the usual three feet to as many as twenty or thirty feet.

DAY SEVEN: Review all that you have experienced and learned this week. Set aside an extra 14 minutes during the day to meditate on the Seven Sacred Symbols and open your heart with gratitude to their healing power.

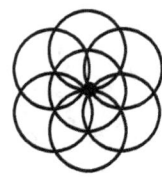

𝒴our 𝒻orehead 𝒫ortal of 𝒫ower
Week Four
Opening to Wisdom and Serenity

𝒫rayer of 𝒫rotection
"Wisdom is mine and I know. Serenity fills my days and nights."

This week will be a time of rest, a time for digestion and assimilation. All you need do each day is spend an extra 14 minutes meditating on the seven Sacred Symbols.

As you spend this extra time each day this week in meditation allow the Sacred Symbols themselves to work for you. You need not do anything but look at them. The rest will be done for you, for you will be using these times as prayerful invitations for the acquisition of true Wisdom and Serenity..

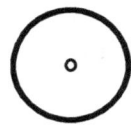 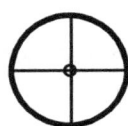 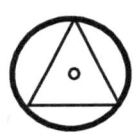 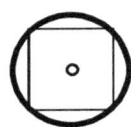  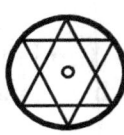 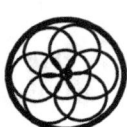

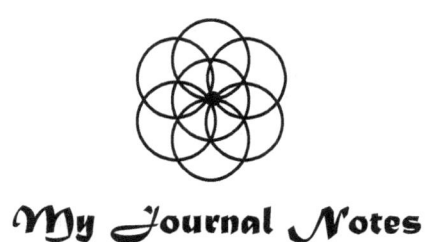

My Journal Notes

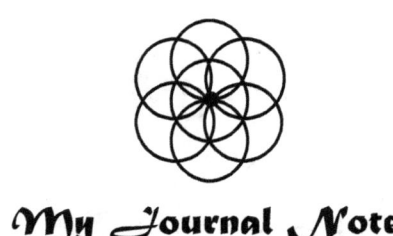

My Journal Notes

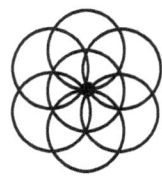

Your Crown Portal of Power
Week One
Opening to Revelation and Your Body

Prayer of Protection for the next four weeks:
"I am ready for God to be revealed. All is Spirit."

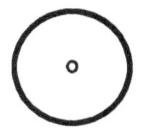 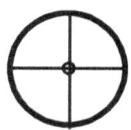 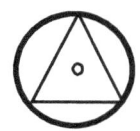 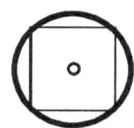  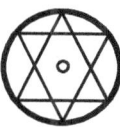 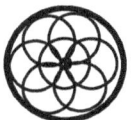

DAY ONE: Affirm throughout the day, "I wish to find God."

DAY TWO: Find time to spend 10-15 minutes to quiet the mind. Visualize the Sacred Cobra, the divine kundalini energy of life, dancing and weaving up the inner channel of your subtle body.

DAY THREE: As your day unfolds, hold the image of the Sacred Cobra resting on the top of your head.

DAY FOUR: Set aside 10-15 minutes of quiet time today, this time visualizing both your physical and subtle bodies disappearing in a radiant stream that enters through your Crown Portal of Power.

DAY FIVE: Spend some time today in a natural environment. Hold the image of the Earth pulsating in time with the Sacred Cobra's dance within your inner channel.

DAY SIX: Set aside at least 5 minutes every hour to reach inward as you affirm, "I am within the Body of God. We are One."

DAY SEVEN: Review all that you have experienced and learned this week. Set aside an extra 14 minutes during the day to meditate on the Seven Sacred Symbols and open your heart with gratitude to their healing power.

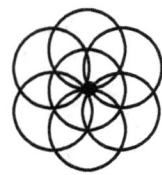

Your Crown Portal of Power
Week Two
Opening to Revelation and Your Relationships

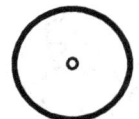 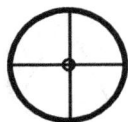 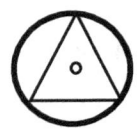 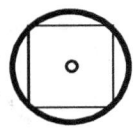  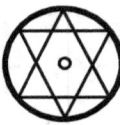 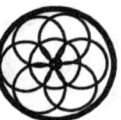

DAY ONE: Affirm throughout the day, "I wish to find God!"

DAY TWO: Refer to your list of relationships or create a new one. Write next to each name, "You are One with God."

DAY THREE: As your day unfolds offer each person you meet this prayer, "God is a part of you. I am honored to be in your presence."

DAY FOUR: Set aside 10-15 minutes to quiet your mind. Then allow your past relationships to flow through your mind. Offer each one this prayer, "You are a part of God. I honor your memory."

DAY FIVE: Awaken earlier than usual today and sit quietly in the silence making this request, "I am ready for God to be revealed." And so it will be!

DAY SIX: As your day unfolds affirm, "I am walking within the Light of God's Love." Hold this image and visualize the Light infusing your whole world.

DAY SEVEN: Review all that you have experienced and learned this week. Set aside an extra 14 minutes during the day to meditate on the Seven Sacred Symbols and open your heart with gratitude to their healing power.

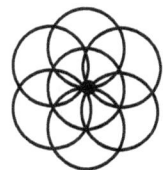

Your Crown Portal of Power
Week Three
Opening to Revelation and Your Mind

Prayer of Protection
"I am ready for God to be revealed. All is Spirit."

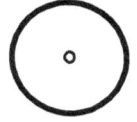 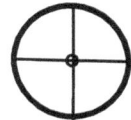 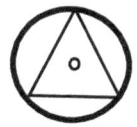 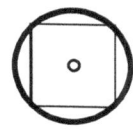  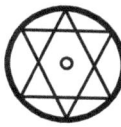 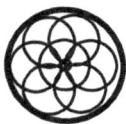

DAY ONE: Affirm throughout the day, "I wish to find God."

DAY TWO: Spend 5 minutes several times today reaching inward and affirming, "God's Mind and my mind are One."

DAY THREE: Throughout the day hold the image of rays of white light pouring into the top of your head, filling your mind and shining out into the world.

DAY FOUR: Throughout the day hold the image of God's Mind filling the Universe with the Radiance of Love so that all forms and divisions disappear.

DAY FIVE: Set aside 10-15 minutes to quiet your mind. As you do offer this prayer, "All is Mind and All is God."

DAY SIX: Throughout the day offer this prayer to the Universe, "Our Minds are joined in God's Mind. God is revealed to us."

DAY SEVEN: Review all that you have experienced and learned this week. Set aside an extra 14 minutes during the day to meditate on the Seven Sacred Symbols and open your heart with gratitude to their healing power.

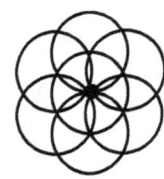

Your Crown Portal of Power
Final Week
Opening to Revelation and Spirit

Prayer of Protection
"I am ready for God to be revealed. All is Spirit."

This week will be a time of rest, a time for digestion and assimilation. All you need do each day is spend an extra 14 minutes meditating on the seven Sacred Symbols.

As you spend this extra time each day this week in meditation allow the Sacred Symbols themselves to work for you. You need not do anything but look at them. The rest will be done for you, for you will be using these times as prayerful invitations for the Spirit to be revealed..

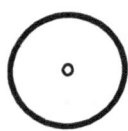 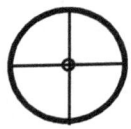 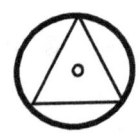 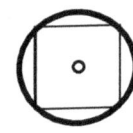  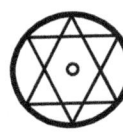 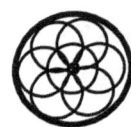

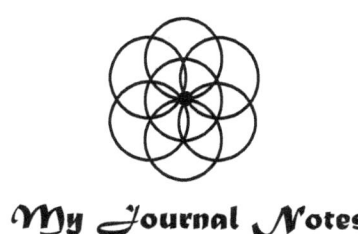

My Journal Notes

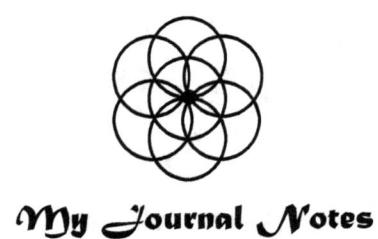

My Journal Notes

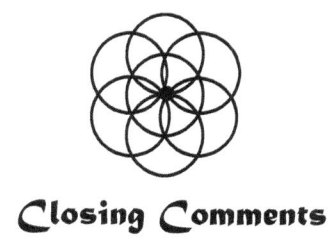

Closing Comments

Dear One,

You have heard the call of Life and have followed Its compelling request. You traveled along the path of awakening for the last months by allowing these daily lessons to open, cleanse and release the Wisdom of the Universe through your Portals of Power and into your world. You are no longer the same person you were when you began.

You have evolved greatly and through your own growth you have helped accelerate the whole world's progress. Both the demonstration of your evolving life and the power that has flowed from you has touched the world, and the world is grateful.

Though many choices appear before you, they are really but one - accelerate your Soul's progress. The insights you have gained over this past year have become more ingrained in your heart and mind than you can imagine. You have learned and you have progressed. You cannot go back to what was before.

Many options for spiritual study and discipline are available. Follow that which calls to you. You may wish to repeat this Workbook again, and perhaps again. This will be good and will only help to reinforce the learning already accomplished and lift you to a higher level of experience and understanding.

Your Soul evolves in a spiraling movement. As you deal successfully with Life lessons, you are spun to a yet higher level of learning. Again and again you learn to open and listen and follow Life as you spiral higher and higher toward transcendence. This is the rhythm of your journey.

I am honored to have served you. Through this program our paths have converged and become less steep and difficult for us both, for we have shared together. May Life fill your Soul with Its love. . .

.. . And may your Soul's progress be swift!

Bette Jean Cundiff

"And then everything you made will be forgotten, the good and bad, the false and the true. For as Heaven and earth become one, even the real world will vanish from your sight. The end of the world is not its destruction, but its translation into Heaven."
A Course in Miracles

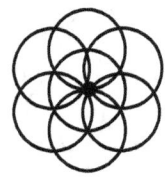

Other books by Bette Jean Cundiff

(* these books include a Spanish translation)

Side by Side – the Twelve Steps and A Course in Miracles *

Hand in Hand – Recovery and Miracles

For children:

The internationally recognized children's Course in Miracle,

original title, "The Children's Material" is now:

Book 1 – Little Lamb's Big Book (for young children) *

Book 2 – Help is On the Way! (for preteens) *

also

Pack Rat's Christmas Surprise *

Mystery at the Everything Exchange

For more about these internationally loved and acclaimed books, go to:

www.miracleexperiences.blogspot.com